Marshall's Journey

The Power of Understanding Alzheimer's

by

Vailia Dennis

First published by AuthorHouse 05/14/04

ISBN: 1-4184-1669-X (e-book)
ISBN: 1-4184-1670-3 (Paperback)

Library of Congress Control Number: 2003099495

Printed in the United States of America
Bloomington, IN

This book is printed on acid free paper.

MARSHALL'S JOURNEY

I have asked myself many times, why did I need to write this book? I wrote because the words poured out of my mind and demanded to be put on paper. As my understanding grew, I knew that I had discovered skills that would help my brother and me survive the painful devastation of Alzheimer's disease. I needed to share these ideas with others in the hope that it would bring them comfort. I know that it can never be easy, but it can be easier. It can never be less than demanding, but it can become more tolerable. This book carries the reader through the decline of a loved one and the thoughtful care given by the one who loves.

Vailia Dennis

CHAPTER ONE

The Beginning

It's difficult to know when my brother's illness really began. In retrospect, I realize this terrible disease must have started many years ago and that I had no way of recognizing it then. I simply believed Marshall had stopped liking and respecting me. Though never physically violent, he was often sarcastic and angry. There were many times that I felt I could no longer live with him, I also knew I never would leave him. It was a difficult period in our lives and the thought of Alzheimer's crossed my mind. With four known cases in our family and Marshall's radical change in personality, I secretly lived with the fear that my brother was becoming a victim.

We had been living together since I retired in 1984, when I left my job in central California and returned to San Diego to make a home for my father and brother. The two bachelors were living in an apartment, eating every dinner out, had the grayest underwear and towels I'd ever seen, and little or no outside activity. My brother was working for an automobile agency and our elderly father still worked two days a week selling shoes. Both had been caring and supportive of me all my life; I now felt it was my turn to care for them.

We rented a comfortable three-bedroom home in a lovely area that was perfect for our needs: one story so that Dad did not have to climb stairs, a wonderful master suite that offered Marshall the privacy he needed, and a bedroom for me that I could dress up with soft white laces that would delight my granddaughters when they came to visit.

Three years later our father died and Marshall and I were left alone. For several years our normal closeness made living together pleasant. He is four years younger and I had always adored my baby brother. As the only two siblings, we shared a lot of our lives, though our personalities were vastly different. He had always been reclusive and I loved being with friends, working with organizations, writing, painting, designing. He was content to stay home, while I needed outside activities. In spite of our differences somehow we had always been compatible.

Then in 1991 Marshall entered the hospital for his second open-heart surgery. The surgery was a frightful experience. He required five by-pass procedures and once again, a valve replacement. Initially the operation seemed to go fine - until he began bleeding internally and the incision needed to be re-opened. Because of the continuous bleeding and the subsequent swelling the doctors were unable to close the incision. There he lay in Intensive Care; kept alive by machines, with his exposed heart covered only by a sterile plastic pad. Eight days later, with the help of many specialists, the incision could be closed and the machines removed. Then began the slow road to recovery. After his forty-two days in the hospital, I was able to bring him home. He was unable to swallow, painfully thin, and very confused.

As time went on he seemed to recover completely, but could not work any longer and without hobbies, interests, or friends he began relying more heavily upon me. Though Marshall had always a loner, he was now becoming a true recluse. He kept himself confined to the house with only an occasional dinner out or a rare visit to a family function. Looking back, I wonder if this was the beginning of his affliction. I began to recognize a change in Marshall's behavior. He became sullen, angry and resentful. He didn't like my going out, did not want any of my friends to visit and would go into his bedroom if anyone arrived. He seemed to dislike me, my cooking and my interests. I didn't understand then; I do now. The terrible disease was slowly taking my brother from me and all that I realized at the time was that I felt hurt and rejected.

The only interest Marshall had during that period was our Shetland Sheepdog, Finian. The dog was more than an interest. It had become an obsession. Marshall's days were spent brushing, feeding, petting his dog. At night the two of them would retire to his bedroom and watch television. When Marshall turned the lights off, Finian would crawl up beside him and they would sleep. Then tragedy struck. Finian was diagnosed with rectal cancer and we had to end his pain. We took him to the veterinarian three times, brought him home twice, then finally had to leave him to be put to sleep. After that loss the two of us cried and Marshall finally declared, "No more dogs in this house. I'll never go through this again." I complied with his decision until, a few months after losing Finian, it occurred to me that Marshall might become more involved and content if we had a dog.

One morning Sunday morning, while he was calmly reading the Sunday paper, I said to him, "Marshall, you are 77 years old and I am 81, what makes you think that we can outlive a dog? I'm going to get a Sheltie."

"If you bring home a dog," he protested, "it will be your responsibility. You'll have to feed it, pick up after it and take it to the vets. I'll have nothing to do with it." Knowing his love of animals I realized that this threat meant very little. I could safely go about finding the right dog for our home.

I found Nicky, a 5 month old sable Sheltie. I arranged with the breeder that if anything happened to Marshall and me, she would take Nicky back and care for him. Then I brought Nicky home. Bringing that puppy into our house was the best thing I could have done for my brother. They spent time together, took little walks in our backyard and often napped with Marshall in the recliner and Nicky on the floor beside his chair. He became Marshall's only joy and interest.

CHAPTER TWO

Recalling the First Stage

I don't know when Marshall's illness really began. Was it when he decided that he didn't want to eat or drink any longer? Was it when he weighed only 119 pounds and became so malnourished and dehydrated that I had to rush him to the hospital? Perhaps it became most obvious that something was mentally wrong when he again entered the hospital in 1994 to have a shunt inserted in the urethra. He had been troubled with urinary problems for some time and suffered bladder infections frequently. This procedure was to help correct the chronic problem.

After the procedure was complete, the doctor placed Marshall in the hospital for overnight observation. I remained with him until late evening. After assuring myself that he was all right, I returned home to feed Nicky and to get some rest. I had no sooner opened the door than the phone rang. It was Marshall saying, "Come and get me. You've got to get me out of here. I just pulled out all the things in my arm (the intravenous) and I'm bleeding all over the bed." I immediately called the nurse, explaining that I was only a few minutes away and would be there at once. Would she please take care of him until I arrived?

It was after that incident that his behavior in the hospital became very strange. He refused to keep any garments on, tore the sheets off the bed and imagined people and animals were in his room. His physician was concerned and decided to place Marshall in an adjoining convalescent home to monitor his condition. During Marshall's stay there a psychiatric evaluation was scheduled.

With the result of that evaluation, I realized that my fears for my brother were well founded. The diagnosis was dementia or Alzheimer's. Now I understood why my brother was so unkind to me, why he said hurtful things and why he complained about everything I did. It was not me - nor was it Marshall. It was the terrible disease. It caused his fear and frustration, his plight of realizing that something was wrong and his not being able to comprehend what was happening. He did not want to be where he was and could not find comfort and familiarity anywhere else, not even at home. Strange things would happen to him there and he could only rebel against the confusion and fear with more confusion and anxiety.

It was when I brought him home that the family and my friends went into complete denial. I felt that if I heard one more time, "But he sounds fine when we talk on the phone," or "He seems to be all right and he looks great," I would scream "You don't understand. He is not all right, you just can't see it." And then the loneliness of the caregive begins. You are alone in the traumatic experience and no one relates to your despair.

How can you expect people, even those who love you, to be supportive if they don't recognize your problem? How can you go to them when you need a hug and assurance to see you through the next unknown challenge? Who offers to stand beside you and be there for you if they don't believe you? And who understands that there are times, in the early stages, that you aren't sure you believe yourself? Can you be imagining this? Maybe it's not really true. Many "maybe's" surface until the next obvious incident and you know you must accept that you're not imagining things: Marshall is very ill.

His acute memory loss became more obvious. He had increased difficulty understanding information, he forgot to pay the bills that had always been his responsibility, and making a decision became perplexing. To eliminate overdue payments, I asked if he wanted me to take over paying the household accounts. He did, and for my very private Marshall, releasing any of his financial information was a totally new condition.

So many things were changing, and change would become constant in our lives. I would have to learn how to handle our new existence and find ways to help him through the difficult times ahead. I would have to become less aware of the caustic remarks and become more aware of his distress. I had very much to learn.

I quickly learned that the things I took for granted no longer applied. His having to make a decision appeared to confuse him, and he became agitated when questioned. It was obvious that I try to avoid that problem. I would no longer ask if he wanted to go for a drive. His answer would most likely be "I don't know," and he really didn't.

So I began my new role of caregiver by simply saying, "Come on, Marshall. Let's take a ride." Usually that worked fine and he would often ask, "Can we take Nicky, too?" We normally could.

Realizing that I could no longer escape the actuality of his condition. I finally had to accept that it really existed and if I was to find a way to handle our lives I needed to seek help.

Help came my way unexpectedly. I saw an invitation in our daily newspaper for caregivers of mentally troubled patients that was being held at a local hotel. The invitation was for lunch and offered lectures by noted authorities. I phoned in my reservation and I now know that it placed me exactly where I needed to be. The first thing that was said invaded my mind and has remained there ever since.

The speaker explained, *"His reality is not your reality. You must get into his reality and go along for the journey."*

During lunch I sat beside Joanne Sala-Di Sesa, a delightful young woman who had a Master's Degree in Clinical Psychology and was working for her doctorate at the San Diego College of Psychiatry. She mentioned that she would soon be facilitating at the college for a group of Alzheimer's caregivers. I anxiously asked if I could become a part of that group. After several interviews, my application was accepted. It became my rock, my place of understanding, my source of growth in knowledge and my much-needed support. Once a month, I was not handling my life alone. Once a month, I was sharing with others like myself and learning and growing with their understanding.

It was during one of our monthly meetings that I learned about respite care. I was becoming increasingly home bound and needed alone time to clear my mind, to feel like my active self rather than a constant custodian. A member of our group informed us that, after having been on the waiting list of the Southern California Caregivers Association for almost a year, he finally was able to receive respite care for twenty hours a month. I applied to the organization and was put on that waiting list. I also applied for assistance from the Alzheimer's Association.

It was a relief to discover that there are many caring organizations ready to help. A great deal of constructive knowledge is available through discussion groups. Books at the public libraries are filled with information, and the librarian will help in finding informative reference books. Knowledgeable people graciously offer assistance through local programs. Caregiver's Association provides seminars, brochures, their own library and limited legal help. Alzheimer's Association also offers the same assistance and I found the brochures they publish to be of exceptional value. There is so much help available. One only needs to ask. I have done a lot of asking, both through organizations and my support group.

At one of our meetings I brought to the group my concern about Marshall continuing to drive. As a whole, they recognized the problem of my taking his car from him, yet they assured me that it was necessary. I realized that, too. But it was such a difficult decision.

Marshall's newest obsession was his car. During the stage of spending money freely Marshall leased a sporty black Chevrolet Cavalier. He loved the car and spent hours cleaning off the last bit of dust from its shining surface and windows. He bought and used many car waxes, tire dressings and other trinkets that helped occupy his time and attention. But it was becoming more obvious that his driving was unsafe.

An incident occurred where he could not identify with the sign that said, "Left Turn Yields." I silently thanked God for the driver of the oncoming car, who stopped short of hitting us. There were other incidents that indicated that his sense of distance had changed. He began driving too close to the car ahead and on one occasion waited too long to come to a stop at a red light. He rear-ended the car in front of him, causing no damage but making me realize that the time had really come to remove his car.

That is when the question loomed before me. "How am I going to accomplish this and save him the pain of losing his car, and his independence?"

CHAPTER THREE

November 2000

The Beginning of the Journal

November 7th

The first stage has passed and we entered the second some time ago. It's hard to tell when the next stage actually occurs. The stages seem to overlap and you don't realize that something has changed. Not until it becomes very obvious that there has been a definite emotional and physical decline.

Marshall's first, or mild stage, involved short term memory loss, hiding objects or simply misplacing them, repetition of conversation, anxiety, confusion and a decided change in personality. I have been told that the second stage lasts longer and escalates the first stage symptoms while adding depression, withdrawal, disorientation and paranoia.

It appears that Marshall has been in this second stage for some time. He has become much more dependent. I now need to make decisions for him and assist him with his more childlike behavior, as I return to the mother-sister role that began that long-ago day in Chicago, where he was born.

I distinctly remember February 13th 1923, when Dad held my hand and led me across the path of a snow-laden square to enter the hospital door. I was almost four years old and my little girl heart was filled with excitement. Something very wonderful had happened that day and I could hardly wait to go up the elevator to my mother's room. A woman entered the elevator with us and as we ascended she asked me, "Where are you going, little girl?"

"I am going to see my baby," I replied. "Mommy had him for me today." That moment began my life long maternal relationship with my brother. Marshall was my baby. Mother gave him to me in many ways, even telling the family who came to visit that they were to ask me if they could see my baby. Mother was the Mommy, but Mommy worked and was gone all day. I assumed the role of protector and guardian for my baby brother. Has anything changed?

November 11th

I know that Marshall must stop driving. I also realize that it might make our relationship more difficult if he believes that I am the one who is responsible for taking his car from him.

Removing his car will be particularly difficult for Marshall. His intense need for independence is involved with his ability to drive. Until now he has been able to hold on to that independence by taking short trips to the grocery or the bank. That also helps him retain his dignity. Because I know him so well, I'm afraid that losing his car might cause Marshall to become angry and resentful. It could then be possible that he would refuse to accept my care.

I decided to phone his doctor. "Dr. Joswig," I said, "I need your help. Marshall's driving has become a real concern. He is no longer a safe driver, however I cannot be the one responsible for taking his license and his car from him. Could you handle that for me?"

"Of course," he replied, "bring him in."

I also asked if I could bring along a tape recorder, explaining that no matter who the culprit was that caused his loss, he would most likely blame me. I received Dr. Joswig's approval. Then I told Marshall that he had a doctor's appointment and we left for Dr. Joswig's office.

Marshall was sitting on the examining table, waiting for the doctor to entered the room. He looked especially handsome, wearing new beige slacks, a beige and white printed shirt and his silver gray hair still showing signs of curl as it brushed back from his forehead. He also looked so vulnerable

His soft brown eyes brightened as Dr. Joswig entered the room and shook his hand. The doctor was carrying a letter that he held up for Marshall to see.

"Marshall," he said. "This is a letter to the DMV. It says Marshall Goodfriend." He hesitated. "We both know him, don't we?" he asked, looking at Marshall and smiling.

With humor, Marshall answered, "I like that sound."

Dr. Joswig continued, "He's a uniformly nice guy and a popular guy. This letter is dated today. It say's Dear Marshall." He hesitated, "Here I am reading it to you, out loud and in person, as we speak."

Marshall chuckled and my heart went cold. He didn't know what was coming; I did.

Dr. Joswig went on, "It says, "Dear Marshall, please do not drive."

Marshall uttered a sad, "Ahhh."

"I consider his driving to be unsafe due to his medical condition. Signed, Dr. Joswig."

He looked at Marshall. "Okay, Marshall?" he asked gently, sympathy showing in his concerned expression. Marshall answered, "Okay"

Dr. Joswig explained, "It's really in your own best interest. We don't want anything bad to happen to you."

Then, to lighten the blow, he handled it with, "Turn the car in, Marshall. Make some money. Get rich. Win the lottery. Invest in Microsoft stock. Take a cruise." Marshall chuckled again as Dr. Joswig shook his hand, and we left the office.

Somehow, I don't think that Marshall completely absorbed what was being said. He had shown no emotion while we were with the doctor, but as we drove home his hands were clenched in his lap and his mouth was set in a tight thin line.

"Do I have to give up the car?" he asked.

"I'm afraid so, Darling," I replied

"Who said so?" he questioned

"Dr. Joswig. Don't you remember? He explained it to you."

"I don't remember," he replied, and sat quietly all the way home.

I have needed the tape several times today and will probably have to continue its use until he accepts that he can no longer drive. He is hurt, but not angry. I feel so badly for him. He has actually lost the most vital proof of his independence that has always been such a strong part of his life. Today began the road to total dependency.

November 16th

Marshall's morning began with extreme agitation. He desperately needed his sister. "Where is she?" "Why doesn't she come home?" "Maybe she's hurt or sick," he said and began pacing about the house while explaining that they have always been close, that this is not like her, that maybe he did something to make her mad at him.

"Your sister's just fine," I told him, "I talked to her on the phone. She's with her daughter Robin. Do you remember Robin?"

"I'm not sure," he answered. How could he not remember the little girl that he helped me raise? Why would I even mentally question that? The simple answer is that he can not.

"Robin needs your sister to help with the children," I explained to him. "You know she has six children with special needs that she's raising. That's a lot of hard work. Robin can't do it alone. The girl that's been helping her had to leave, so your sister is staying with Robin until they can get new help."

"She didn't tell me that," he argued. "She always tells me where she's going and when she'll be back. I don't remember her telling me anything. Maybe she's sick or something."

No amount of explaining helped. I phoned a member of the Alzheimer's group whose wife is similarly troubled. I asked, "What do you do?" and he answered, "I lie a lot." A flash of understanding. *"His reality is not my reality."*

I hung up the phone and turned to explain to Marshall that I had to run to the grocery for a loaf of bread and would be right back. "I won't be long." I said, "Take care of Nicky while I'm gone. Don't let him go outside."

"I won't," he said, as he looked down at the puppy lying beside his chair. They would both be fine for the few minutes my task would take.

I hurriedly drove out of the garage and around the corner, where I parked. Then I picked up my cell phone, called home and said in a high, gay voice, "Hi, Honey."

He answered, "Thank God, Thank God," and there were tears in my eyes.

After reassuring him that I was all right, that I would have to stay with Robin for a couple of weeks and that I loved him very much, I drove home.

His face was bright and smiling as I opened the door. "My sister just called." he said, "She's all right. She'll come home soon."

He was at peace. The frustration and anguish was gone and he was ready to relax in the recliner, watch the same news that played constantly all day and drink his Ensure. We were back to whatever our "Normal" is.

November 18th

Insuring that Marshall is properly nourished has been a real challenge. He rebels at all food, though it is interesting that he wants to sit at the dinner table in the evening, put his napkin in his lap and wait for me to serve dinner. He will take only two bites and firmly state that he doesn't want anymore. It's frustrating for me to prepare food that will not be eaten. But I do understand his need for a routine to keep his life as normal as possible.

I prepare simple dishes and later serve him an Ensure. I've been working on the problem for a while and believe that it now has been solved with the Ensure shakes I prepare for him three times a day. The Ensure, with three large scoops of ice cream, is whipped in a blender. I add a banana to one shake for potassium and Metamucil to the last shake.

I have been told that ice cream is considered a fluid, so the combination appears to answer all of his physical needs.

November 19th

I have been grieving the loss of my brother, knowing that he really is lost to me. No longer even short returns to the present. I was still silly enough to answer his question, "Have you seen my sister?" with the answer "I am your sister." I brought out a picture of me and found that it made no connection in his mind and I suddenly understood why.

Though I am doing well in spite of the age, I do have white hair and wrinkles and a body that has shrunk three inches. It is impossible for him to recognize me when in his mind he sees the much younger, more physically attractive sister of many years ago. So I now must remain "That Lady."

Chapter Three

Today has been a very difficult day. He doesn't understand where he is or where he lives. "I think I'll go home now" is said quite often. I believe that home is in Mission Hills, a residential area of San Diego, where we had lived for so many years. It was a large, two-story 1930's home where, as a single mother, I raised my children with my family filling in and spoiling them.

Their Uncle Buddy (Marshall's nickname) had always been their most involved father figure. He taught my son, Bruce, the art of deep-sea fishing and helped my small daughter, Robin, learn to catch a baseball. He playfully teased them with his wry sense of humor. His "Go to bed, Robin" or "Go to bed, Bruce," became an inside family joke. At any time, under any condition, he would tell them to go to bed and I never understood whether it was when they were getting the best of him or he was getting the best of them. But many giggles and laughs came after those words and no one ever went to bed.

Marshall insisted that the children and I save money through the school year, so we could go on a summer vacation. Because he never told us where we were going, our vacations became real adventures. He would take us to the Redwoods, or the Winchester House, or to Yellowstone National Park. He was the most wonderful and patient traveling companion. My children dearly loved their Uncle Buddy. They still do. Precious memories today contributed to my sense of loss.

November 21st

I'm still fighting for his sanity. I began reading anything I could find about Marshall's condition. I now know that I must stop fighting for his understanding. To do that, I will need help. First, I called the Alzheimer's Association and asked for additional literature. Then I went to the Library and brought home books on dementia and Alzheimer's. It will take me time to absorb all that I need to know.

I opened a page of a book that explained Alzheimer's victims have a fear of shadows, they can lead to hallucinations. That explains the hall and bedroom lights that he leaves on all the time. I didn't understand why he did it, especially since he was the one who used to insist that we keep lights off to reduce electricity costs. "Do you have stock in the Electric Company?" he'd scold, as he walked through the house turning off any unnecessary lights.

I will no longer follow him and turn off the hall and bedroom lights. There is no need for night shadows to be added to his fears.

November 22nd

Today we kept his doctor's appointment for a routine checkup and a prescription for Aricept, a medication to help Alzheimer's patients. I stopped to have the prescription filled so I could start giving it to him tomorrow morning. Marshall's mood was even worse when we returned home. "What am I doing here?" he asked. "I want to go home."

Somehow the appointment seemed to agitate him. "Buddy," I said, "I'm sorry, Dear, but we can't go home. We rented the house to some other people, but when they move out, I promise we'll go home." He seemed content with that.

Trying to convince him that he is home is of no avail. Although he has been living in this house for seventeen years, going to bed in the same room all those nights and eating his meals at the same table, it would not be an idea that he could accept. I suddenly realize that he really does not live in this time span. His whole mental picture of his life is possibly thirty or forty years ago. Nothing will bring him to the present. Marshall doesn't live here anymore.

I believe that it is important to write in this journal that I am not a Pollyanna. I know anger, despair, impatience, confusion - almost every negative feeling one may have. I also know that no one benefits from my allowing any of them to become evident. My agitation contributes to his agitation. Should I become irritable, he can only respond with irritability or fear. He doesn't really understand what is happening and that is when the fear sets in. I must work at maintaining a steady calm for him and actually, for my own sanity.

November 23rd - Thanksgiving Day

Family members phoned to invite us for dinner, but Marshall refused. He used his incontinence as an excuse. It became clear that he could not identify with the holiday and I felt all right about staying home with him. My granddaughter, the "other Vailia" who is such a special part of my life, joined us.

She's very loving and kind with her Uncle Buddy, and with me. She and I have a very close relationship. Through all the turmoil in my life, her entering the door of my home brings a moment of joy. So today she entered, kissed Marshall and, while brightly talking to both of us, began helping me prepare our Thanksgiving dinner. It was a small festive version of the traditional meal, with candles glowing and the best china shining on the yellow tablecloth. Marshall ate very little, but seemed to enjoy our celebration.

November 24th

My son, Bruce, arrived to spend a few days with Marshall and me. He was here less than two hours before he asked, "How long has this been going on?" His expression was shocked and unbelieving.

"I've been trying to tell you about it during our phone calls," I replied. Then realized that my telephone calls could not have made Bruce aware. The condition must be witnessed to be understood, and the loneliness sets in with the lack of support from family members and friends who don't understand.

Eventually, you come to realize that they simply can't relate to your fears and frustrations because they haven't been exposed to the cause. Many of them live in denial. Just as I did when my mother's sister, Sadie, became afflicted.   I eventually saw her in a fetal position, wearing a diaper and mentally destroyed. I didn't realize what my beloved Aunt had to go through before reaching that last horrible state. I didn't understand the terror that filled her earlier days. Today I do know and there are times that I feel despair when I realize what lies ahead for Marshall

November 26th

The Aricept is not working. Marshall has had adverse reactions to the drug. He is much more confused and having hallucinations. He asked who that strange woman was that was wandering around the house. He later felt that he had just seen our cousin, Warren, and had a nice talk with him. Warren has been dead for three years, also an Alzheimer's victim.

Marshall is pale, agitated and seems to be frightened to the extent that he is locking every door and window, and pulling the blinds shut against the outdoor light. I phoned Dr. Joswig's office and explained that Marshall needed to be withdrawn from the medication. They agreed. I hope that Marshall will return to his previous state. It was not a good state, but certainly better and less frightening than what he is facing now.

November 27th

Today is the day that I said to myself, "Okay, I give up. I completely surrender." Just as I can't stop a wave from coming in from the sea, I can't stop what is happening to my brother. I can't make it go away. I can't control it. I can't make him understand that I am his sister, that he lives in this house, that he needs to wear a nighttime undergarment, that his next doctor's visit is two weeks away no matter how often he asks. Despite controlling, explaining, losing patience, trying strength, despite everything I have done, the wave still keeps coming and it will always come, and now I finally accept that what I must do is join his journey, and it is a lonely journey.

Marshall is with me, but I am alone. He can no longer contribute to our relationship. He can no longer do small tasks like emptying the dishwasher or taking the trash to the container just outside the kitchen door. He doesn't know where familiar things are, can't find the light switch or the silverware drawer. He wants to go home, wants his sister, is truly lost and I don't understand why my heart isn't broken.

November 28th

Today he got dressed and wanted to find a bus to take him to San Diego. He needed to get in touch with his family. I couldn't help him because I am no longer a family member. I am "That Lady,"

He needed to see someone but couldn't remember the name. To ease his tension I took him for a walk at the shopping mall. Diversion helps. We walked a while and shared a sandwich at the food court. Driving home he asked, "I don't have to go to that lady's apartment, do I?

"No, Dear," I said, and then I asked, "Is there something wrong with that lady?" I needed to know if I was doing something that might be uncomfortable for him.

"No," he replied, "She's a nice lady. But I'm not sure. I think she wants me to be her beau."

I often kiss my brother goodnight, or give him a hug or a pat on his shoulder. In spite of the humor of his reply I asked myself, "what do I do now?" I know he needs to be touched, needs to feel secure and loved.

So I replied "Well! We're not going there. We're going back to our house." At home I will do as I have always done. Keep loving him and showing it.

Marshall then said, "Maybe I should call her (That Lady) and tell her that I'm not coming?" He settled for waiting until tomorrow to phone.

He was calmer, but stayed up later after we got home. He obviously needed companionship, to be listened to. It helps him, but as he goes to bed later many nights, I lose more and more of my independent time.

Chapter Three

November 30th

In the evening he's in Mexico and can't get home. He is with "Lady" but needs to get back to San Diego, back to his family. He desperately needs his family. To distract him, I said "Come on, Buddy," I said. "Let's take a walk with Nicky. He would just love to go for a walk."

"Okay," he said, "but then I want to go home."

"We will," I replied, and picked up Nicky's leash as we headed out the door. Our walks are very short. Marshall can only shuffle slowly, so walking around the corner and back is enough for him.

Nicky does not enjoy the walks and becomes excited when we near home. "Look," I said as Nicky began to pull toward the house, "Our silly Nicky doesn't want to walk anymore. He wants to go home now. Are you ready to go home?"

"Yes," a tired Marshall replied, and once more we could inside and settle down for the evening.

Later I called our cousin Gail to make arrangements for a short visit to her home. It is really important to help him understand that his family is close and loves him. I'll drive him over as soon as she makes arrangements. I realize that my efforts can only be temporary solutions, but necessary. I'm certain that he will be more at ease if he stays in contact with family members.

It's also necessary that I add solutions to my own medical problems. I have begun struggling with Angioedema. It's an allergic condition related to hives. My lips and eyes swell and there are deep red welts all over my upper legs and stomach. The doctors now, after testing for all possible allergic reactions and finding no cause, have prescribed anxiety medication. Perhaps stress and anxiety are the cause.

Strange, when I answered all the anxiety questions on the test that came with the medication, I found that only one applied. "Do you feel Fatigue?" Could I feel anything else?

CHAPTER FOUR

December 2000

December 2nd

Can a caregiver be aware of their patient's decline on a daily basis? No. One day you wake up to the fact that he no longer knows how to handle a toothbrush. Another time you become aware that he cannot tie his shoelaces or put the shoes on the right feet. Looking ahead it seems that his condition is advancing rapidly. Looking back you realize that he has been losing his mental ability for some time. The loss seems to be moving more rapidly now as his condition worsens. One thing that I know for certain is that the primary emotion he lives with is fear.

Fear is a creator. It never stands alone. It creates flight, anxiety, confusion, anger, helplessness and despair. It is easy to recognize all these reactions when caring for an Alzheimer's patient. But all I could see initially were the results. Seldom was I able to recognize fear as the source of his problems until I understood that it really existed. Though I now know that eliminating all his fears is an impossible task, recognizing and softening the impact is the best I am able to do.

I have found ways to comfort Marshall by accepting that he lives in a world that existed many years ago and that he is frightened when he can't find his way back. He doesn't live in this house, I am not his sister, his mother and father are still alive, his new puppy is Finian, our last Sheltie, not Nicky. The fear surfaces because he really doesn't know where he is, doesn't know who you are, is afraid of the dark, of being left alone, of feeling that something is terribly wrong, but unable to identify the strangeness that he lives with daily.

Understanding his fear is the only way to cope with the things that disturb him. I cannot bring him back to the present, but I can join him and help with the lost soul that he has become. It is not a simple task. That is where creative thinking becomes important.

Today Marshall approached me with his toiletries in his hand. "I think I'll take these upstairs and put them in my room," he said.

An uninformed caregiver might remark, "Marshall, there is no upstairs. Go put them back." Then the fear sets in. "Why doesn't she know there's an upstairs?" or "Why am I thinking this way. I know there's an upstairs and I need to go there". Creative thinking allowed me to say, "I'm sorry, Honey, but you can't go upstairs any longer. Dr. Joswig doesn't want you to climb stairs because of your heart condition."

"Oh," he said, "that's right. I forgot about that. I'll put them back." I watched as he left me to return his toiletries to his room. My once proud and handsome brother is now a bent gray-haired old man who shuffles as he slowly walks away. He seems so tiny and so very fragile.

There can be many answers to a situation like that. A stair might "be broken" and have to be repaired. The stairway may be "too dark" because a bulb has burned out. Whatever the reason, he will soon forget what he wanted to do and because the fear has been eliminated his life can become peaceful once again.

December 3rd

As I was getting him ready for bed this evening he insisted that there are others who sleep in his room, too. He was sure that a man and woman had been there all day and they sleep in his other twin bed, but he couldn't identify them. I explained to him that if they were making him uncomfortable I would get rid of them.

"How will you do that?" he asked.

"I'll kick them out," I said. "I'll take away their key and tell them that if they come back again I'll call the police."

"Good," he answered and settled comfortably in his bed.

I placed his covers over him and gently stroked back his hair as I assured him that he was safe, that I would always be with him. Then turning his nightlights on, I closed his bedroom door, so that Nicky could not disturb him, and went into the family room to sit quietly in the recliner and reflect that I now know what the "Caring" in Caregiver means.

Chapter Four

December 4th

I've discovered that I cannot write daily in this journal. Marshall's need for my attention intensifies. I will just have to try to record the paths of our lives as often as I can.

December 6th

I face a recurring problem that has existed since Marshall was diagnosed with Alzheimer's. Family, support group members, and personal friends all have asked the same question. "Does Marshall know that he has Alzheimer's?" That question is one that many families must face.

My conclusion has been, "No. And it's important that he doesn't know."

My answer brings about various opinions and I find myself needing to qualify my decision and feeling annoyed by the firm statements of "He needs to be told."

I silently ask, "Why?"

I have tried to explain that there are two reasons I am not telling my brother of his condition. One is that he is too familiar with the progress of the disease and would readily understand

39

what the future holds for him. He spent many days, visiting with and caring for our Alzheimer's afflicted aunt. He watched the magnificent mind and body deteriorate until all that was left was a small skeleton lying in a fetal position in a crib. He suffered with her through her fears and her decline, and he would not be able to bear the thought of having to face the same fate. I cannot find any reason for him to receive information that would bring more anguish into his life.

The other reason is that Marshall was not diagnosed early enough to make rational decisions. As for an estate that would require consideration, he will have little to leave. No home that he owns, no property to consider, no life insurance that would possibly need to be adjusted. Even his car is leased and can be returned to the dealership. His investments are in both our names and are not large enough to warrant any legal assistance. He has no great decisions to make and I see no point in causing him any alarm.

I've discussed the problem with Dr. Joswig and accept his opinion that Marshall's illness does not need a name, it just exists.

Chapter Four

December 8th

Marshall accepts his hallucinations as real. I have to accept that, also. Trying to explain to him that his delusions, or hallucinations, do not exist can be counter-productive. He may easily become very agitated and alarmed when he is the only one seeing or hearing whatever it is he sees or hears.

Because I have heard that certain illnesses, medications or infections might induce hallucinations and delusions, I contacted his doctor's office to make sure that no physical condition was creating his problem. After finding that was not the case, I started researching through the brochures and books that I have on hand. I need to know how to cope with this condition. I discovered that what he needs is for me to calmly let him know that I understand and will take care of the alarming situations. It reassures him when I recognize his fears.

While researching I also discovered another idea that applies to his behavior, and a cause that I never considered. Delusions can manifest as wrongful suspicions that Marshall shows toward others who come into our home, or to me. I had considered it a form of paranoia that seemed to occur when he hides or misplaces an object and cannot find it. What I discovered was that his inability to locate the object may become too difficult for him to

41

accept. It is easier to imagine a theft as the way to explain the loss. So now I agree that someone must have taken his wallet and that we will just have to get a new one. I also reassure him that the person is no longer in the house, so we won't have to worry about it any longer.

Distraction may sometimes help when he is frightened by a hallucination. He recently saw a strange black dog lying on the floor of the family room. To distract him, I suggested, "Let's go into the kitchen and have a little dish of ice cream. We'll take care of the dog later." That helped, especially since ice cream is his favorite snack. When we returned to the family room he no longer saw the dog. These situations do not occur often, but when they do acknowledging his fears may remove what could become very disturbing encounters.

There is some disagreement as to whether my method of handling delusions and hallucinations is the accepted method. There is the opinion that not recognizing hallucinations or delusions may be more correct.

I have no medical background. I'm just a loving caretaker who has discovered what works best for her patient. Staying in his world with him seems best for both of us. Most importantly, it is working. He looks to me when he is frightened and is satisfied that I understand and will help him.

December 11th

The lost wallets now concern me. Without a wallet Marshall has no identification on him. Should he wander or have an accident, no one would be able to locate where he lives or know what medication he is taking. Because he is on Coumadin, that is especially alarming. He needs the medication for his heart condition, but it thins the blood so dramatically that a small cut can cause excessive bleeding.

In searching the yellow pages under "Medical Supplies" I found the answer. Because this is the weekend, I will have to wait until Monday to order the form that must be sent for his Medic Alert bracelet. I think that I will order two, at least one is certain to be lost.

Marshall does not yet wander, but he may, and being lost would be terrible for him. Once he has the bracelet he can be safely returned home. I keep trying to find ways to eliminate his fears. Some I can handle, others I cannot and I desperately wish I could.

December 12th

Today I seemed to focus on the changes in my life. I became aware of the things that I have had to give up. Not resentful, just aware, just part of the life that I am now living.

A well run, neat home: I consider myself a "Neat-nick," which to me means everything in its place. That provides me with a sense of beauty and allows me to look at a room and find it warm and inviting. Not that I have been spotlessly clean. There's often been dust around, but even the dust had its place on top of tables and buffets. Sometimes there are things that get thrown into drawers, but again, they're in the right drawers. So the ten minutes I used to take to straighten the house before I went to bed have now become twenty and it's too late to put away the slippers, robe, flashlight and gloves that lie on the floor of the family room. He's asleep and I wouldn't dream of waking him. I'll just wait until morning and put all the many out-of-place things where they belong. That is if I have time to do it in the morning.

An active social life: I can't attend my organization meetings that take place on Tuesdays and Thursdays. I haven't received any respite care yet. In fact, until I am able to obtain the help that I need for a little out-of-the-house time by myself, I can't have lunch with friends, go to a movie or simply drive to the mall and window shop. Though I have no social life right now the lack is interesting in that it weeds out the acquaintances from the friends. The phone doesn't ring as often as it did, but when it does you know that it is someone calling who really cares. There is real gratitude for the relationship of family and friends that phone and share their time with you.

Having his help: All the little things that he used to do that I must do myself. Taking out the rubbish, emptying the dishwasher, running down to the grocery for a loaf of bread, picking up the cleaning, fixing his own breakfast, cleaning off the dinner table, putting gas in the car. Each one alone is a small thing, combined they add much to my responsibilities.

Privacy: That's a big one. Quiet times for myself are almost nonexistent now. Originally, he was in bed by nine. That allowed me a few hours to do things like writing in this journal, speaking on the phone and just having fun with my computer. Now he is up much later. By the time I have helped him with his night protective underwear and pajamas, and tucked him into bed, I am too tired to begin any project. There are times that I am followed to the bathroom or he is at my bedroom door as I try to dress. I often have interruptions when I am on the phone and many questions about my private conversations.

Fortunately for both of us, I understand his need to be near me. I represent his only emotional and physical security. Although we have discussed the same things many times, he must communicate. It has become his only means of being alive in this world. Someone must hear his concerns and his thoughts, someone must answer his fears, someone must care, and that someone must be me.

December 14th

I received his Medic Alert bracelet today. It contained all the required information, except for his name. How could that possibly be acceptable? It seemed to me that the most important fact, in the case of his being lost, would be that someone could call him by name. Without that capability his fear might not be alleviated.

I phoned the company and they explained that his name, "Marshall Goodfriend." was too long for the space. I then suggested that they redo the bracelet with the name "Buddy Goodfriend." That will work and he responds to Buddy as well. Buddy has been his nickname since childhood. It began with me being called Sis and him being called Buddy. The Sis got lost, the Buddy remains.

Chapter Four

December 15th

A wonderful day. I will now have some relief from being home bound. But from two organizations, not just one. I called early this morning to speak with Ann, at the Caregivers Association, because I have been feeling pretty confined and needed some relief.

"Could you please tell me where I am on the waiting list?" I asked.

She replied, "It's interesting that you called. You have arrived at the top of the list and I was just in the process of arranging help for you."

That was great news, though I must admit some trepidation about leaving Marshall with a stranger. Nonetheless, It was delightful to know that I would soon be receiving twenty hours a month to do with as I pleased.

Shortly after speaking with Ann, I received a phone call from Carla. She was calling from the Alzheimer's Association to inform me that she had found a volunteer to assist me with respite care for sixteen hours a month. Does the good and the bad and the in-between always come in bunches?

Of course I was pleased, but I had to be fair and explain to Carla that I had just received twenty hours of respite care from the Caregiver's Association.

"That's great." she said, "Many people have both. It's really no problem."

"Really?" I replied with delight. This was much more than I expected, but I still felt it necessary to inform Ann of my sudden windfall, and to know that it was all right with her organization.

"Of course," she said, "many people have both." Exactly the same words I had heard previously and I relaxed with the pleasant thought that I am really going to have some time to breathe alone and feel free.

December 19th

Ann Sanderson of the Caregivers Association arrived today. She came to interview Marshall and me, and to make certain that our household qualified for the program. I enjoyed her visit. She's a charming young woman who sweetly expressed friendship and concern. I found myself liking her very much and hoping that we could stay in contact with each other. She explained the program and what was being offered. It was to be respite care from a qualified assistant that would be sent to our home from an agency. The association would pay for ninety percent of the cost and I would be responsible for the balance.

How wonderful! This was not a volunteer, but someone capable of really assisting Marshall with his needs. She might perform light housekeeping tasks, could do the laundry and be capable of calming his anxiety while I am away. I feel so good about this arrangement. Hope Marshall will be comfortable, too.

December 20th

My first day of respite relief. Darlene, a volunteer from the Caregivers Association, arrived at noon and I had four splendid hours to do with as I pleased. Well! not exactly four hours. It took more than half an hour to make Darlene and Marshall comfortable with each other. Then I needed to prepare his Ensure and make sure that he drank it all. I also found a video movie that I thought they might both enjoy and finally left, after giving Darlene my cell phone number with the instructions that should he become anxious, she was to call me. I would either speak to him on the phone or return home.

It was the first time in months that I had been out of house by myself and as I drove away I wondered what I was to do with my special time. The truth is that I needed to go to the bank, and the grocery, and the cleaners. I wanted to stop at the library and pick up a new book-on-tape for listening enjoyment as I drove around. I had some things that should be returned. Of course, I might stop for lunch but that could take too much time.

I know that I could take Marshall with me to accomplish some of those chores, but that is really difficult. I have always moved rapidly. Marshall's steps are incredibly slow as we walk down the aisles of a market. I accomplish so much more when I am alone. So I wasted my precious time today by handling chores. Next time I will make an effort to do something pleasant for myself.

December 21st

I usually turn to my computer after Marshall is in bed. He most likely will get up at least once to make sure that I am here. So I stay awake until I am certain that he has settled down for the night and write at my computer until my eyes want to close.

Tonight I am reflecting about the importance of my meetings with the Alzheimer's Support Group. My appreciation is a little about-face. I've always been somewhat gregarious and certainly independent. My many years in the world of business brought that about. So when I decided to join a support group it was out of desperation. The "Me" that thought I was strong enough to handle everything on her own, couldn't believe that talking to a group of people would solve anything. Still, I didn't know where I was going, what I was doing, or how to handle the upheavals that were taking place in our lives.

I felt that no one else was living my situation, and I was certain that no one close to me knew anymore than I did. Well! the members of a support group don't know much more either, but together we share and learn and grow, and that means that I now look forward to the fellowship and the constructive ideas that I find there. I handle my life better, I handle Marshall's life better after being exposed to the friendship and support the group provides.

December 23rd

The holidays are upon us and I have squeezed in everything that I could do to make them festive. That really is important only to me. Marshall has never been enthusiastic about celebrations. Only for my birthday. Then he has been wonderful. Normally, he couldn't wait for the day to arrive and would approach me a couple of weeks before my birthday on April 11th to tell me of his suggestions for my gift.

Most exciting was one Sunday morning when he sat drinking his breakfast coffee and said, "I've thought of three things for your birthday. We can go to the mall and you can buy whatever you want at your favorite store, or we can have a brunch at the Inn and invite the family and friends, or I think I can still get a ticket for you to attend the Baryshnikov Gala and Ballet."

Of course, the decision was instant, but I was concerned about the cost. "I would love to go to the ballet," I said, "but I know it will be expensive. At least a hundred dollars." He assured me that it was all right and did not let me know it cost more than two hundred dollars to attend that special evening.

Baryshnikov dancing Giselle was exquisite and I did stand next to him at the Gala. That birthday gift is my most memorable. Is it any wonder that I choose to do whatever I can for this very special brother.

December 24th

A day to celebrate. Adrianne arrived today. She is an Alzheimer's volunteer and will come to stay with Marshall every Saturday for four hours. Adrianne is a single mom who works during the week and can only provide respite time for me in the evenings or on the weekends.

I will not ask her to come most evenings because it is then that Marshall is at his worst. It seems that "Sundown Syndrome" is a recognized condition that causes the patient more insecurity, fear, anxiety and becomes present for many at nightfall. That is the time that Marshall is most troubled and needs the comfort of my being with him. However, there are a few special occasions during the year when I will leave him at night.

Six evenings a year I attend the La Jolla Playhouse with my cousin, Hymie. On those nights I make sure that I have my cell phone with me to call home before the play and during intermission. It does not satisfy him completely, but seems to help a little. He is awake when I return home and will then take the Ensure that he refused earlier, along with his nighttime medication. Three evenings a year, I go to the Opera with my granddaughter, Vailia. That is especially wonderful. But those are the only times that I leave him at after dark.

It really doesn't bother me to stay home with him at night. It is only during the day that I am aware of being homebound, and even unable to go grocery shopping by myself. I have tried taking Marshall with me. That, too, is difficult. Though he holds on to the cart when I take him with me, he does not understand that he needs to push instead of pull, and I find myself pushing both him and the cart. Bad back effort.

December 25th

A strange holiday. I realize that I've done very few of my usual holiday activities. I've not made lovely wreaths or centerpieces to give to my friends. I've not baked the special Hungarian pastries that my children have always looked forward to at this time of year. Perhaps the most important thing is that I've sent no cards to those I care so much about. The cards we have received are lined up on shelves in our entertainment center and I look at them with both the joy of having friends and family remember us, and regret that I have neglected so many very special people.

December 26th

There has been a definite change in Marshall. He no longer fights about putting on an overnight pad or taking a shower. He is softer and his natural sweetness is more evident. As I watch him move into the deeper stage of the disease, another thought comes to mind. I wonder if there is a possibility that the violence that you hear about regarding Alzheimer's patients, may not be somewhat induced by the caregiver's inability to recognize where the victim is and what his needs are emotionally.

There seems to be so much frustration for Marshall when he

is being corrected for what he says or does. He is unable to make a choice or follow an instruction. He doesn't know what he wants or why he should change his underpants more often. Bedtime is any time he feels bored, even though it may be only six o'clock in the evening. Demanding, coaxing, insisting, all cause more frustration and fear, which in turn may cause violence.

There still appears to be some remaining thoughts of "What is wrong with me?" "I don't know who she is." "I don't know where I am." The other night when I tucked him into bed, he asked, "What if I'm left alone all night. How will I know where to go?" I calmed him by stroking his hair while letting him know that I would never leave him alone at night; that I will always be there when he wakes in the morning. He is very insecure and needs reassurance.

I am certain that each caregiver has his or her unique situation. For me, I continue to search for understanding and a deeper level of patience. I need to draw on that to help me get through the rough spots. Most important, if I can maintain the proper attitude, it may help him remain peaceful and calm. People who are understood, who can remain peaceful and calm, are seldom the same people who respond with anger and violence.

December 27th

I'm still not always as aware as I should be. Sometimes I forget and expect reasoning to reach his brain. I often explain too much. I have learned that short and concise sentences are all that he may be able to absorb and if it is necessary to repeat a statement, the exact words must be used to avoid mental confusion for him. But there are times that I feel some annoyance that I cannot make him understand what is usually a simple concept.

Today I was tired and felt cranky. I tried to make Marshall understand that we needed the backyard door open slightly so that Nicky could get in and out. Though it probably frightened Marshall to have the door open, I was torn between his needs and that of the dog.

I decided to bring Nicky in and only leave the door open when Marshall is not in the room. But there are times that I think I have to make too many concessions and it occasionally annoys me. Still, in spite of the strain, I also know that nothing can change the path I have chosen. He has no path. It is as though he has been dropped in the middle of a sea with no shore to reach. Just dog-paddling to stay afloat and one day to melt into the warm water again.

December 28th

Today my cousin Hymie came to relieve me for a few hours. While I was in the room Marshall asked her if she had talked to his sister. She answered, "Yes, I have and she is just fine." Later he did not know Hymie, but said that her name was familiar and confused her with Robin.

I know that it is difficult for the family members who love him not to have him recognize them. But the family is being wonderful now and continues to try answering him in an appropriate manner. That means that they too must get into his reality and communicate on his level. I sent them the following letter to help them understand him and his needs.

Dear Loved Ones....

Both Marshall and I eagerly look forward to your visits. I do understand that it may be a little difficult for you to relate to a Marshall that you no longer know. Perhaps what I am writing to you may help.

First: Marshall may not recognize you. That is because Marshall no longer lives in this time frame. He is living back at a time when you were very young, and he cannot relate to the person you've become. It is interesting that he still loves you, wants to be near his family, and would probably know who you are if you could remove thirty or forty years from your appearance. I can't, so he no longer knows me either.

Second: Because Marshall is living in a different period it may help if you can try to go there too with your answers. He may ask about his mother or father, and expect that you have recently seen them. This part is difficult, I know. We all will just do the best we can.

Third: In some delightful way, Marshall retains his sense of humor, so he will respond to light or funny remarks, and probably add a few of his own.

The Marshall that we have always known is gone. The Marshall who remains will still respond to your love and caring with warmth and love of his own.

Our extended family brings stability to both Marshall and me. There have been many times that our cousins have called to take us out to dinner. It's been so special to have Gail and Mark phone and ask, "Can you be free for dinner this Tuesday night?" Or a call from Hymie and Steve suggesting that we have dinner with them next week. Hymie and Gail have often come themselves to take us to dinner and share time with us. Every visit, every dinner, every kind gesture they have made has been a blessing for Marshall and me.

Once in a while, Marshall will ask one of them if they have seen his sister. They give him an answer while I sit there and wish he could know that I'm his sister. It's not that it hurts me, his not knowing. I understand that. It is just that I can't take away his pain of missing her.

CHAPTER FIVE

January 2001

January 3rd

Marshall is incontinent. It was a problem long before I realized that there was no solution and little ability for control. He was and would remain incontinent. The wet beds, the constant rushing to the bathroom, the soiled trousers, all would continue to be difficult to deal with.

Changing the bedding has presented a special concern for me because I have severe back injuries. Osteoporosis has caused several fractured vertebrae and combined with arthritis has the potential for extreme pain. I'm fortunate that I have a high pain tolerance and, when that is added to determination, it is not likely that I will stop doing whatever I feel is necessary.

Over-the-counter pain medication helps keep my back pain tolerable. It seems to work as long as I don't bend over for prolonged periods of time (like changing his bed). It's odd that I never realized how much bending and lifting was required for that simple task. But it does increase the pain, so I decided to begin the search for ways to make it easier.

Discussing Marshall's incontinence with his doctor resulted in a prescription for Detrol. That is the medication that should assist in controlling bladder spasms. It may help with the constant urgency that makes leaving the house difficult and it might save Marshall the embarrassment of wetting through his clothing.

He has always been meticulous about himself and his surroundings. For that reason I am now also concerned that the urine odor he occasionally carries about him will permeate his room. I can make certain it doesn't happen by laundering his clothing, but keeping his mattresses free of absorbing the odor, or of permanently staining, requires some other type of treatment.

Chapter Five

The solution began with a trip to a local store that brought about plastic mattress covers to protect both twin beds. The covers seemed to me to be uncomfortable to sleep on. So I found plump mattress pads to go over them and solved that problem. At the same time a thought occurred to me. When in a hospital the entire bed is not changed, only a half sheet is spread over the area of wetting. That brought about another solution. I purchased disposable waterproof pads, then spread a half sheet over the one that I laid on his bed. I tucked the sheet in tightly so it would remain secure through the night. I will have less to handle in the morning and I should be able to do it without pain. The bed preparation, along with the protective underwear that I help him with at night, may allow him to stay drier and more comfortable.

It really is necessary to help Marshall do things for himself and I try to give him only as much assistance as he needs. I don't want to take from him anything he can still do. My effort is to have him retain as much independence and self-respect as possible. So I keep looking for answers. One idea that I thought might make it easier for him was when I discovered that pull-on protective underpants are available. They're slightly more costly, but because they are so much like his jockey shorts, he may be able to use them during the day.

While I was gathering the items for his room another revelation appeared. I was suddenly aware that Marshall might have more than one reason for not recognizing me as his sister. There are many times he is completely nude. His nudity occurs when I have to assist him with his shower or help put on the night underwear that he can't fasten because of the tabs. My very modest brother seems to be able to handle that help comfortably with a caregiver. I don't believe he could with his sister.

January 4th

Words and thoughts are getting much harder for him to express. This evening, after having gone to the bathroom, Marshall came into the kitchen where I was doing the dinner dishes. He looked distressed as he stood in the doorway. A deep frown furrowed his brow as he said, "Something is wrong in my room."

"What is it?" I asked.

"It's white and round and floating around. It has something to do with urination."

I couldn't understand what he was trying to say. "What does it do to urination?" I asked.

"It makes it go faster or slower," was the reply.

He was getting upset, and again I couldn't relate. "Come, Dear" I said, "let's go into your room and you can show me."

I followed him and we went into his bathroom. I thought something may have fallen in the toilet and was floating around. Nothing was out of place. It was then that he said, "It's in here," and headed for the bedroom. I followed him and watched as he went directly to the floor fan that was still running. Of course! It was white and round and floating around. Poor darling, he could not use the word "fan." He could not remember how to turn it off. His distress this time was not fear, it was his sense of helplessness.

January 7th

This morning we again faced a re-occurring bedwetting problem. His bedding, including blanket and spread, was soaked with urine. I've tried saying, "I know that you can't help wetting the bed, and that's all right. But when you do, Dear, please don't make it up. Just throw back all of your covers and I'll take care of it."

Sometimes he does but there are times he doesn't, and I find a surprise when I prepare his bed at night to discover that I have to make a complete change. Though frustrating, I realize that it is hard for him not to make up his bed. He has been doing that every morning of his life since he was a small boy. My asking him to change his 70 year old habit is unreasonable, but I keep hoping that one day he can handle it and make it easier for both of us.

Still, in spite of the problems that we face during the day and evening, we always kiss each other goodnight and I leave him with "Sleep good, Buddy. I'll see you in the morning," and make certain to remind him that I will always be in the house with him all night. I hope that satisfies him and that he doesn't wake again to come out and see if I'm really here.

January 11th

I had no help today and found myself short of grocery items and especially needed to pick up Marshall's prescriptions. My only solution was to take him and Nicky with me. Marshall rebelled at first. He wanted to stay home because "My sister may call." After my patiently telling him that she could not because she was working, he consented.

The three of us sat in the front seat where Nicky put his head on my knee while we pulled out of the garage, but soon turned toward Marshall and laid across his lap. I heard Marshall quietly whisper, "That's my sweetheart," as he softly stroked the puppy. I could leave them for a short period of time while I ran into the store for the things I needed. Marshall would not leave Nicky alone in the car, so I felt they were both safe.

He is very protective and involved with his dog and often asks, "When I go home can I take Nicky with me?" And I answer, "Of course."

January 15th

I believe that there may be an advantage to being an older caregiver. Marshall reaps the benefits of my regrets. Since everything appears to have a plus and minus, the plus of my age is the wisdom I have gained from experience, the minus is having much less strength caused by an aging body. I suppose you just have to balance the two. But when weighing on the scale of life, I try to let wisdom weigh a little more. To this day I regret that I didn't have that wisdom when I cared for my aging father.

I dearly loved my father. He was a pixie of a man who even in old age dressed smartly, had a sparkle in his eye and was aware of every female that came near. He charmed them when he called them "Honey" and flattered them with his attention. All very innocent and all delightful. He often wore a little brown corduroy hat with a jaunty feather on the side, and I teasingly called him my "Leprechaun".

Dad aged beautifully and really didn't begin fading until he reached his 85th birthday. That is when the repetition began. Most annoying were the hours he spent going over his personal mail again and again. Then he would wait for me to return from work to discuss the same mail that we had discussed the day before, and the day before that.

As I opened the door in the evening he would be standing there with mail in his hand asking me, "What do I do about this. I don't know what it means."

"Dad," I would say impatiently, "We've already taken care of that. I'll go over it with you again after we've had dinner. Right now there are other things that I have to do."

That was true. Fixing dinner for him and Marshall, doing the dishes, answering the important messages that I had not been able to receive, all demanded my immediate attention. What I didn't realize then was, so did he, as he turned and quietly walked back into his room with the mail in his hand.

Chapter Five

My father died when he was 90 years old. I truly regret the times when I was too impatient to recognize his need. I became acutely aware of what that need was when several months after his passing I was listening to a doctor on my car radio. A woman phoned complaining about the same condition with her aging mother. The doctor explained that it was her mother's fear of death that kept her involved with reviewing letters and bills. It helped her keep in the present and away from the fear.

How I wish I had known that when my father needed my understanding. I do now and both Marshall and I benefit from my having the knowledge to look beneath the action and find the source.

January 20th

Not being his sister is my most difficult problem. Especially when his need for her becomes so strong that he begins wanting to phone family and friends to find out if she is with them. This is not a subject to argue about. He really cannot recognize me as his sister. No amount of my reassurance that she will phone, or come home soon, eases his need to be with her.

Tonight he insisted upon calling my friend, Alice.   He was convinced that Vailia was with her.   There was no way I could distract him. Knowing that was so, I dialed Alice's phone number for him. I silently prayed that she could handle the situation because there had been no time to prepare her for his questions. Blessed Alice ended their conversation in tears. She recognized his despair and wept for the Marshall she had known. As he hung up he handed me the phone and said, "Thank You. You're a nice lady."

Every night he asks about his sister and every night it is painful to know how much he despairs that she has not come home. It is difficult for me not to be able to ease that pain. I am helpless against his feeling of being abandoned by me, and I am helpless against finding any way to make it easier for both of us. Not all the love and tenderness I feel for him can help him know that I am here with him.

January 24th

Today went pretty well. Marshall seemed content much of the time. He petted Nicky, watched his news channel, dozed a few times in the recliner and then, at about 4:00 o'clock this afternoon asked, "How about going out for dinner?"

We had gone out for dinner at least once a week for years. Marshall seemed to enjoy the change and I loved the times that

I didn't have to cook and clean up the kitchen. We only stopped dining out about a month ago, after we had eaten at our favorite Chinese restaurant. That evening we ordered two cups of hot and sour soup and Marshall's favorite entrée, a mixture of vegetables, shrimp, beef and chicken. He ate a little of the soup, two of the shrimp and declared that was enough. Much of the dinner was packed to go. Neither of us think it tastes as good the following day, so it eventually gets thrown out. But now he is asking again to eat dinner out and I am very hesitant.

Because he eats so little, my first silent reaction to Marshall's question was "It's such a waste. He won't eat but a few bites. We're just wasting money." On the other hand (I reminded myself of Tevye in Fiddler on the Roof), on the other hand "He's thinking of doing something different. He may just want to get out of the house and that's all right. He may not eat, but he may enjoy the outing. Waste or not, it's the right thing to do."

"How does going to Marie Callenders sound?" I asked. "You've always enjoyed their cream of potato soup."

"That's fine," he answered. He was pleased. His eyes brightened and he seemed to be more alert.

"All right," I said, satisfied with myself and my decision. "I've just a few things to do here in the house. Then I'll get dressed and we'll leave for an early dinner."

It's interesting that many restaurants are considerate of the elderly and their smaller appetites. My appetite certainly has diminished, and Marshall's is almost non-existent. To share our order is the answer and most restaurants, including Marie Callenders, allow sharing.

We sat in a comfortable booth and I ordered a cup of the soup for each of us. They serve it with corn bread and honey butter so it becomes a fairly hearty entrée. I ate all of mine. Marshall ate about half of his. I told myself not to worry, Ensure would take care of that later.

"How about a dessert?" I asked when we had finished the soup.

"I don't know," he answered. That is the common answer for him now.

"They have great pies. Would you like your favorite cherry pie?"

"That sounds good."

Still bright, still smiling at the waitress, he said. "I think we'll have cherry pie."

"Good choice," I said.

I then asked the waitress if she could divide a piece of cherry pie in the kitchen for us and add a little ice cream.

"No problem," she said, and returned shortly with our pie half-slices and a full scoop of ice cream on each plate.

"That's very nice of you," Marshall said as he looked at our plates

He ate part of the pie, all of the ice cream and seemed very satisfied with our outing. I'll never hesitate again. Whenever he asks, we will go out for dinner.

A problem frequently occurs when we are in a restaurant. Marshall visibly looks as normal as any other diner, but often becomes uncomfortable when the waiter questions him about our order. He really can't make that kind of decision and becomes distressed simply because he can't.

I've solved that. I have taken an old Library card that looks somewhat like a credit card and written a note on the back. It says, "My brother is ill. Please address all your questions to me. Thank you." I then hand it to the waiter before placing our order. Marshall questioned me about it tonight. I simply replied, "It's only my credit card, Honey. I made a mistake and gave it to her too soon."

"Oh," he answered, and that ended his concern. When the waitress brought our dessert, she sweetly smiled at Marshall as she placed it before him and said, "I know you'll enjoy this." Once again I became aware that most people are kind and willing to be helpful.

January 27th

Why did it take me so long to understand that Marshall's brain could not accept more than one step at a time? Yesterday I ask him to put on his underwear, his shirt and his pants. I found him trying to put his underpants on over his head and realized that he could not absorb the multiple instructions.

Today I tried saying, "Buddy, put on your socks," and I waited.

"Put on your shirt," and I waited. "Now put on your pants." That worked fine and neither of us felt frustrated or irritable.

January 30th

It has become clear that everything is hesitant for him. The speed in which he used to pick up a fork or drink a glass of water has changed. Because his thought processes are slower, his actions require more time. It is obvious that Marshall's brain has become more damaged and there is no way to hurry him. Attempting to do so only results in his becoming agitated.

That is sometimes difficult for me. I'm a get-things-done person and waiting to accomplish the next task can prove annoying. Obviously, the solution must be mine. It cannot be his. So doing the dishes or taking clothes out of the dryer may have to wait as I sit with him while he slowly drinks his Ensure.

Again I need to reach for a deeper level of patience. I need to understand that there will be less accomplished in a day, that our lives will move more slowly and that I must be satisfied in knowing that what I am accomplishing is being my brother's caregiver. But I really do hate seeing dirty dishes waiting on the kitchen counter.

CHAPTER SIX

February 2001

February 2nd

Robin arrived from Arizona this morning. Though it is not easy for her to leave David and the children, she has been very worried about her Uncle Buddy and felt that she needed to see him. The fact that he may not recognize her has become a real concern. She's often asked, "Mom, if I came out there do you think that he'll know me?"

I had to truthfully answer, "Darling, I don't know. He still may, but not all the time." That was the best I could offer.

During our phone conversations I had been trying to prepare Robin for Marshall's decline. Not only mentally, but also physically. He has shrunk several inches and now only stands 5'4" tall. The shrinkage has caused his stomach to extend and his shoulders to bend forward. Behind his glasses, the bright brown eyes that sparkled with wit, now lay quiet and insensitive. He no longer looks like the Marshall we've always known. But then again, I don't look like his sister either.

I've paralleled him in many ways. I have also shrunk several inches, my stomach extends and I don't walk as straight as I did. Age has caught up with my appearance. I must admit that I resent all the new wrinkles that seem to appear daily on the skin that had been so smooth just two years ago. It was fun to be eighty years old and have people think that I was sixty-five. Now the stress and excessive weight loss has added the missing years and my ego is suffering.

When Robin entered the house today she found Marshall withdrawn and less concerned about what was going on about him. She saw a weak old man sitting in a recliner, eyes too blank to really comprehend anything. She hurried over to him and kissed his cheek. "Hi, Uncle Buddy," she said. "It's me, Robin."

"Oh," he replied, and continued to stare at the television.

She stood stunned for a minute and then hurried past me and out of the room. I quickly followed her and found her sobbing. Through her tears she said, "I want my Uncle Buddy back." I replied, "So do I," and my eyes filled with tears, too.

I put my arms around her and held her close as I said, "Darling, it's alright to cry. But let me explain. I know you think you've completely lost your Uncle Buddy. You have to know that somewhere inside him still remains the man who has always loved you. Be patient. He will recognize you occasionally. What he needs from you now is to have you treat him as you always have, with love, acceptance and understanding. He has always given you his unconditional love. Now he needs the same from you."

Robin walked back to where he was sitting. She sat on the couch facing him and told him about her trip here and her plans of taking him with her to the San Diego County Fair. She reminded him that they had shared the fair together for many years. "Now," she said, "we will share it together again."

He may not have comprehended what she was saying, but he did listen and seemed to be involved. Occasionally he remarked, "That's nice," and she would smile at him and go on.

There were a few times today that he did recognize her and was happy that she was here. With each recognition it was as though she had just arrived and he greeted her warmly. He was even able to ask about David and their children. But there were others periods when he became confused. Then he believed that she was our cousin, Hymie, or asked about the strange woman who was staying in our house.

"Is she going to be here all the time?" he asked me.

"No, Dear. She's Robin and she's come to stay with us for a little while. She loves you very much and remembers all the wonderful things that you did for her when she was a little girl. Do you remember when you took her and Bruce to Yosemite and we saw that funny little bear sitting on a fence?"

"No," was the reply.

"Well," I replied, "you did that for us, and when a big bear came near our car you told us to close up the windows quickly.

We did, and we watched the bear through the glass until it went away. That was a wonderful vacation and you planned it all. You did a great job." He smiled at that and seemed more comfortable that Robin had come and was a part of our family.

February 3rd

Robin decided to take Marshall and me out for brunch today. The restaurant we went to is very special. It's located at our beautiful historic Rancho Bernardo Inn. The restaurant and terrace overlook a rolling green golf course and a beautiful valley peppered by tall trees and homes with terra-cotta roofs that glow in the sunlight. We ate on the terrace under an umbrella that shaded us from the sun and allowed a warm balmy breeze to envelope us. A February day in San Diego can be unbelievably perfect; today was. I prepared a plate for Marshall (an interruption as I'm typing. He is standing at the door of my computer room asking how I'm doing, but really checking to make sure I'm here. "I'm doing fine,' I answer him, "I just have to finish some work on the computer and I'll be with you.")

He left and I'll go on. At the restaurant I placed the food that he usually likes on his plate. He seemed to be uninvolved and ate little. (Again an interruption with the question, "So where are you heading?" "Nowhere, Dear, I'm staying right here," I reply "Oh!

I thought you were going out.")

I'll stop now and go into the family room with him. It's becoming very obvious that at night he becomes more needy. As he moves farther away, his fears and insecurities continue to escalate. He seems to need constant reassurance that our lives are intact and I will always be near him. (Marshall at the door again, "Will you be here in the morning?" Once again I answer with the same words, "Of course, I am always here. I will never leave you alone.")

That doesn't register for any period of time, but satisfies his immediate need. It also is obvious that I must find another time to write.

February 7th

Robin made arrangements to meet our cousins Hymie and Gail for lunch in the restaurant at Balboa Park. The park is a special part of our city and from the time my children were small we spent our days there, visiting the museums, having picnics near the fountain or lunch at our very special restaurant. That is where my daughter, who is now a grandmother, celebrated her ninth birthday. It is where Robin and Bruce would join me for dinner before attending musical performances at the outdoor Starlight

Bowl. Understanding Robin's desire to return to the park, and the restaurant, is simple. Both are filled with wonderful memories.

I originally felt that I could leave Marshall once again with Adrianne. But he came to my room while I was dressing and looked so distressed. His face was pale and the forlorn look of his bent head made me realize that he might be feeling frightened and neglected. I decided that he was too upset to leave with anyone. I called Adrianne and cancelled our appointment. Marshall needed to go with us.

At lunch he participated in nothing, but seemed content just to be there. Once again I ordered what we could divide. Though he didn't eat that either, he had a plate of food and was not isolated from the others. I believe that setting a plate in front of him treats him with consideration and respect, and that is not difficult to do. I remember who he was and honor what is left of him. Keeping that in mind makes my job easier. Looking ahead I know that it will not always be easy to cope. Not easy, but each effort makes me realize that it is better to try than to live in my world without him.

February 8th

I've been busy with Robin. Marshall seemed to resent that I was not solely involved with him. It became evident this morning when he appeared at my bedroom door saying, "There has to be some changes. I need to live somewhere else."

To me it seemed he was saying, "I feel neglected and alone."

In spite of understanding his problem, I was hurt. I have tried so hard and though I recognized his concerns, the statement was painful. Despite my reaction, the problem remained and it had to be resolved. It was then that I recalled what I had said to my young children when they were being unreasonable. So I said the same thing to him.

"Buddy," I said, "that is not an option. This is where you live, and where both you and I will stay. Robin is leaving tomorrow morning and we'll be alone again."

He answered, "Okay," somewhat reluctantly and returned to his television. We'll be all right tomorrow.

February 10th

Robin left today and I miss her already. Not only is Robin my precious daughter, she is also my third arm, the one we all wish we had so we could handle more than two things at a time.

From the moment I took over for the care of my brother, she took over caring for all my medical expenses and health insurance problems. It is done brilliantly and I have no forms to fill out and no battle to fight when my secondary insurance refuses to pay. I don't know how she does it, but I seldom write a check for medical expense.

I often try to express my gratitude. I don't know how I would have handled another responsibility. Especially one that I dislike so much. It may be that my practical side has not been fully developed, but taking care of monthly statements and financial obligations is my most unpleasant chore. Her handling my accounts is truly a blessing.

Now that Robin is gone, Marshall has started focusing on Vailia. "Do you know Vailia Dennis? My sister and I got separated. Why can't I reach her?"

He picked up the morning mail including a book sent by Reader's Digest addressed to Vailia Dennis "We need to send it to Vail," he said. "We will," I answered, and he was satisfied.

Being able to keep him comfortable about his sister's absence is often a challenge. It helped today when I said that she was working in Santa Barbara and would probably call in a day or two. Because Robin has been visiting here, I had to change Vailia's location from Robin's home in Arizona to another. So I explained that Vailia had to return to her old sales territory. That the company she had worked for needed her, but she would call him often and come home as soon as she could.

Those answers are always temporary solutions, but they needed to work today because I now have a more pressing concern. I just realized that Marshall's mouth is in terrible condition. For many years he wore a partial plate. Today I discovered that it has disappeared. No amount of searching produced it. Apparently he has either hidden it so well that it cannot be found or has been thrown it out. No wonder he can't chew or bite into anything.

Because Marshall is a World War II veteran, I thought that I might get help through the Veteran's Administration. When I phoned I found that he is not eligible for their assistance because his problem is not service related.

I will call his HMO tomorrow and see what they have to offer. There must be some answer to the problem.

Chapter Six

February 11th

I phoned Marshall's HMO and received their dental list. I made an appointment for today and was pleased to find that Marshall did not rebel. After X-rays were taken we went into the dentist's office and the dentist explained what needed to be done. All remaining teeth had to be extracted and Marshall would have to wear a full set of dental plates.

That meant that Marshall would have to be put under anesthetic, have teeth extracted, impressions made and learn to tolerate upper and lower plates. His being able to adjust to those procedures was highly unlikely. Recognizing his fears, his impatience and his inability to handle stressful situations, I felt it was impossible to consider this dentist's proposal, but I was curious about the cost.

I decided to ask the dentist how much he would charge if we were to consider the service. The answer was $5,400.00. We live on fixed incomes and could not possibly handle that amount. So the problem still exists and I have to find an acceptable solution.

February 13th

Marshall's 78th birthday. It's a day that I would like to have celebrated, but for Marshall it meant nothing. The gifts he received from me and the children gained very little recognition. He looked at them and slightly shook his head in acceptance. What pleased him most is what I called a Birthday Card shower. It began the week before his birthday when I phoned all the family and many of my friends. I suggested that they might want to send him a card, in fact two or three, and I would do the same. The idea occurred to me when I remembered how much he enjoyed receiving cards before he became ill.

It really worked well and I was delighted to see his pleasure when the cards started arriving and he opened the envelopes. I read the messages written inside while he admired the art on the front of the card. There are many cards in a bright row lining our entertainment center. They helped make his birthday a pleasant day for him. This evening I prepared his favorite dinner of roast brisket and potato pancakes, and was surprised to find that he enjoyed the pancakes. He actually placed three of them on his plate, loaded them with sour cream and appeared to relish his birthday dinner. (I will have to make potato pancakes more often.)

When I helped him get into bed tonight I had the sad thought of wondering how long he would be with me and if this might be the last birthday we two will share.

Chapter Six

February 17th

An impossible day. I was impossible, Marshall was impossible, and I had reached the end of my patience. Dr. Joswig had ordered a bro-time blood test for Marshall in order to check the coagulation of his blood. It is required monthly because he is on blood-thinner medication. After my helping him shower, shave and dress, he firmly declared that he wasn't going to go.

His stubborn chin hardened and there was no way to make him understand that it was necessary. After my explaining that the doctor needed that information to make sure that his blood was not too thin, he insisted, "I'm not going. It's my body and I can do whatever I want with it."

"Buddy," I said, "of course it's your body, but you're not a doctor and you don't always know what is best for you."

"Oh! Yes I do," he answered stubbornly.

"Do you think that you're always right?" I asked angrily. (As I write this I'm thinking, Vailia, where did the patience go?)

"I am always right," he answered.

Mother! She made him always right, and made me always wrong, and I felt it and I flared. "Of course, you're always right. Just as you've always been the good one and I've always been the bad one." I said sarcastically.

I continued with "Our mother did a great job with us."

Was I still jealous of my mother's relationship with my brother? I remember feeling jealousy as a small child. Sometimes it reared its ugly head when he was referred to as the "Angel" of our family. When I grew older I realized that perhaps my being an unwanted child had caused my mother's attitude toward me. I was born to a mother who was much too frightened and much too young.

On the other hand, Marshall was the desired baby, precious and adorable. I had been a skinny sickly little girl with dark circles under her eyes and a Buster-Brown haircut that did little to enhance the straight dark-brown hair. Marshall was a dream. Soft brown eyes that held amazing sweetness and beautiful dark curls that framed a perfect little face. Our personalities were different too. I stood my ground and Marshall was much more compliant.

The bond between my mother and brother lasted all the years

of her life. He adored her and she doted on him. They were each other's best companions and their closeness may be the reason that Marshall never married and had a family of his own. Mother died when Marshall was 43 years old. Perhaps too late for him to seek other relationships. Am I still jealous? Oh! No. But I do understand how we both arrived at who we are today. I am the strong one, he is a more gentle soul and the truth is that I dote on him, too. So, tomorrow we will try again for the test. He won't remember today's problem and I will devise a way to make the test acceptable to him.

I'll probably take him for an afternoon drive, and while we're out I might say, "Buddy, what do you think? It's time for you to go to the lab. Would you like to get it taken care of today so we won't have to bother with it tomorrow?"

Most likely his answer will be "I don't know." But even that will be his decision and he may be more comfortable when we arrive at the laboratory.

He is generally agreeable to the test, so the bro-time problem could be solved. While that is being solved, I will also correct my hasty reactions. I'll just probably always let him be right. It doesn't really matter. I'd rather be kind than be right.

February 20th

I thought that it would be easier to care for Marshall as he declined into the more advanced stages of the disease. I was wrong. The earlier stages when he was fighting to keep his independence, his dignity, his masculinity and his ability to help himself were much easier than his present decline.

He doesn't mind the care I give him when I shave him, help him brush his teeth, put on his pajamas and tuck him into bed. He is no longer angry about the night protective underwear. He only knows that he must be near me at all times and he lives with the fear that I may leave him alone. I understand that the need for constant reassurance of the caregiver's presence is normal for Alzheimer's patients as they progress into advanced stages of the disease.

Not only are my physical efforts more demanding, but emotionally he is more insecure and constantly needs my presence. Yet I am aware that he personally demands so little of me. Just to be near and safe. The efforts that I make, I demand of myself.

Keeping him clean and dressed well, inventing ways to help him feel secure, carrying the load alone and thinking that no one could do as well for him. These are all self-inflicted conditions and I can handle them because they are on my list of "Must Do's."

"Must Do's" are interesting. They became a part of my life many years ago when I lived with my father, brother and grown son. Though I worked daily, I was also the home-maker for these men. That meant that I was responsible for the cleaning, marketing, cooking and keeping a well-run home.

One Saturday, my normal cleaning day, I was in the bathroom doing the nasty job of washing the toilet. I hated that task and felt resentment that it had to be my job. I felt the same way when I changed linens or had to do the laundry.

I suddenly became aware that what I was feeling was resentment and I knew that is often the cause of family discord. I didn't want to go that path. I really don't think that I wanted to change what I needed to do, I just didn't want to feel so annoyed.

"The truth of the matter is," I told myself, "that you will continue to do whatever it is you need to do. So how can you make it more acceptable?"

"Don't think about it," I answered me, and "Must Do's" were born.

A "Must Do" means that I do not allow myself to think about what I'm doing. Instead I can sing a song in my head, I can think of a book I want to write, I can plan my next vacation. I can focus on almost any pleasant thing while comfortably ignoring an unpleasant situation.

"Hurray! for me." I congratulated myself and then amiably went on about my task. That was then, and this is now, and in the now I can revert to my "Must Do" concept while I am caring for Marshall.

My lack of privacy often requires a "Must Do." It is difficult not to feel disturbed when your privacy is constantly being invaded. That occurs in many ways, including my closing the bathroom door to take a shower. It is then that he keeps knocking on the closed door and asking if I'm all right. I know that it's one more expression of his needing the reassurance that I am in the house with him, but it can be very annoying.

I've solved that problem with a timer. This morning I brought it out of the kitchen and set it close to him. Then I said, "Buddy,

I'm going into the bathroom to take a shower and I have to close the door. When this timer goes off, I'll open the door and come out again." I set the timer for a few seconds so he could recognize the sound. Then I reset it for fifteen minutes and closed the bathroom door.

Despite that preparation I still felt uneasy. I found myself not relaxing while I waited for his interruptions. I was focusing on the wrong thing. I stepped into the shower and indulged myself with a song in my head and warm water on my skin.

I relished my fifteen minutes. More wonderful, the timer worked. Marshall was holding it when I approached him. He smiled as I removed it from his hand.

"It hasn't gone off yet," he said.

"I know," I answered. "That's Okay. I just finished a little early."

"Are you going out?" he asked.

"I don't think so," I replied. "But if I do, I'll take you and Nicky with me."

He was relaxed, I was relaxed and I love kitchen gadgets like timers.

February 23rd

For years Marshall read the morning paper. Lately I've found it unopened and lying on the couch. I believe that he no longer is able to read. My first insight was when I left notes for him that I believed would keep him comfortable while I was away. I would print the notes in large letters using a black felt-tip pen. They would tell him where I would be, how to reach me and what time to expect me to return. I'd then tape them to the wall beside the television. They were also useful to those caring for him.

Leaving notes worked for a while and then stopped. That became apparent after I came home several times to find him very upset. He would angrily question about where I had been or why I didn't tell him what time I'd be home. It was obvious that he ignored the notes and refused to accept the information from anyone who was with him. It happened often enough for me to realize that the notes had become useless.

So reading the newspaper no longer fills his morning hours and I am finding it harder to occupy him. He is unable to walk more than short distances. He will ride in the car with Nicky, but soon wants to go home. I've tried taking him to the dog-park where he could watch Nicky at play. The other dogs approaching his dog frightened him and again he wanted to go home. Now there is little left to amuse him. Just a short walk with the dog in the back yard, listening to musical CD's, watching the television and a few video movies.

It has become important to recognize that certain television subjects are best avoided. I wasn't aware of that until a movie showing a severe thunder storm frightened him.

"Look what's happening," he cried. "That's a real bad storm. We'd better get Nicky and get out of here."

I walked over to him, brushed back his hair as he stared up at me with frightened eyes.

"It's alright, Buddy," I said, "it's only the television."

I kept watching him as I walked over to the TV. "Look, Honey" I explained, "It's just the TV. I'll get a different channel. You like this one better anyway." Because he loves animals, I switched to the Discovery Channel.

"Are you all right now?" I asked.

"Yes," he replied, and settled back into his recliner. The incident was gone, but now I need to check to see what he is watching. I find that he does best with sports and animal shows as well as watching the all-day news channel. Even though some things shown on that channel could be alarming, he seems to know that it is the news and is not bothered by them.

February 28th

I have been sad all day today. I'm consciously mourning the loss of my brother. I miss him even as I stand beside this man who doesn't know that I am with him. I can't find Marshall anywhere. Not in looking at his frail little body or his sunken dark eyes or his pale drawn face. Not in listening to the garbled words from a mouth that said so many bright and wonderful things. I want him back and I can't have him back. And it's all so strange to feel like this while he's right here with me.

Bruce called while I was writing this. He phoned to see if his uncle and I were all right.

"Hi! Mom," he said. "How are you doing?"

"Okay," I answered.

"You don't sound okay. What's going on?"

"I'm just feeling very sad today," I replied.

"Are you writing in your book?" he asked.

"I was when you called."

"Read me what you've written."

I read the last chapter. Bruce was quiet for a moment.

"Mom," he then explained, "it's the grieving before the dying. Slowly losing Marshall is still losing him. I know it's awful for you. Writing in your book brings it all into focus. It's understandable - that is when you are more aware of your grief and sadness. I wish there was something I could do to make it easier for you."

"I'll be all right, Honey," I said. And I will be.

While we were talking I had said that I was mourning

Marshall's loss. Bruce called it grief. I asked him what the difference was about the two words and I received the usual Bruce reply.

"Look it up, Mom," he offered. I often wonder if he doesn't know the answer or if this is just his way to make sure that I understand. I've also wondered when the parent-child role reversed. I did look up the two words and I am grieving and I am mourning. The words are interchangeable.

Bruce called it "The grieving before the dying." He was right, but it is a different kind of grieving. It is not the wringing of the hands or the face swollen with tears. It is not holding your body tight and rocking in pain. It lies deep inside, hidden from you and the world around you, while you observe the slow death of a fine mind and a firm body.

Today I allowed myself to indulge in the pain. Tomorrow I will go about my usual routine and bury yesterday's thoughts. Tomorrow the sun will shine in San Diego, the air will smell sweet and Marshall will be here with me.

CHAPTER SEVEN

March 2001

March 1st

I did it. I found a way that we could take care of Marshall's dental problems. After discovering that there are dental groups that operate much like HMOs, I phoned the Dental Association, explained the circumstances and asked if they could refer me to such a group. They supplied me with several names. Checking the yellow pages for a convenient location, I found one that was close to our home. We went to see the facility today and I now realize we can financially function within their costs. They require a nominal amount to join the group and the yearly fee includes Xray's, teeth cleaning and check-up visits. Marshall accepted having the Xray's taken today and we made an appointment to return to see the dentist on March 12th.

There is a negative in joining this dental group. They are extremely busy so there are long periods of waiting between each procedure. That represented an unexpected problem.

We have family jokes about Marshall's lack of patience with long delays. No way do we expect him to wait in line for a movie or for dinner at a restaurant. So I found myself trying to console him with, "Just a little longer, Buddy. They have to develop your Xray's before the doctor can take care of you. It shouldn't be too long now." I tried chatting about little things and brought magazines for us to look at. It helped some, but I could feel his tension and impatience. I shudder to think of how many times we will have to wait. But when the office manager assured us that the total cost for his care will be under $1,000.00, I decided that we can definitely find a way to return for an appointment on the twelfth, and wait.

March 5th

Why do we, the caregivers, neglect ourselves so badly? It

seems to be a common thread that runs between all of us.

My friend, Sharon, who is caring for her very ill husband, fainted yesterday and had to be rushed to emergency. She is now in the hospital and one of the diagnoses is dehydration. Her afflicted husband is not dehydrated, nor is he malnourished or neglected.

We have already lost one of the members of our support group. She was an especially wonderful caregiver for her husband of many years. He became increasingly more difficult with early signs of violence, such as a raised fist or a little shove. During a session she explained that she was troubled about making the decision of putting him in a nursing home or trying to keep him with her a little longer. At the insistence of her children, she placed him in a care facility. That is when she shared with us that her feelings of stress and guilt had become more acute. Last week she died suddenly of a heart attack. It often seems to be true that being a caregiver for an Alzheimer's afflicted person has aptly been titled, "The Fatal Occupation."

The sad fact is that the damaged health of many caregivers exists, and it is not necessary. I must admit that I am guilty and that I excuse myself because I am too busy, too occupied mentally, emotionally and physically, and too tired. That seems to justify the self-abuse.

Today I spoke with my daughter-in-law, Debby, and received a scolding for neglecting to take my morning medications until noon. Marshall always gets his on time, but though I often think about taking mine as I hurry through the morning, I wait until I find the right time. Never realizing that the right time is "Now."

Debby's scolding went like this, "When you travel on an airplane with a small child you are given instructions about the oxygen masks. First, you are told to put one on yourself, then assist the child. The reason is obvious. The adult needs to be capable of helping the child, and you need to take your medications so that you are capable of helping your brother."

Of course she was right. In both cases the reasoning is the same and I must, and will, do better. I will not neglect fluids, I will not neglect proper nourishment and I will take my medication on time. And while I am doing that I will be doing it for my patient as well as for myself.

March 8th

I have seen evidence of Marshall's anger when he responds with clenched jaws working near his temples and a deep frown over glaring dark eyes. It has occurred when I demand more than he can handle or correct an error that he thinks is true.

We go back to *"His reality is not your reality. You must get into his reality and go along for the journey."* Operating from that concept prevents me from expecting too much of Marshall. It also helps me recognize his limited awareness and where his frustration levels lie.

For Marshall the frustration begins when he is being corrected for what he may say or do. He is unable to make a decision or follow a command. He doesn't know what he ate yesterday or why he should change his underwear more often. The confusion appears to remain in thoughts of "What is wrong with me?" "I don't know who she is," "I don't know where I am." "What if I'm left alone all night, how will I know where to go?" Demanding, coaxing, insisting - all cause more anxiety and fear, with fear being the primary emotion.

Marshall's reality is very real for him. I must recognize it and support what he perceives to be true. That doesn't mean that I walk on eggs in caring for him. It only means that I understand where he is and try to follow him. I cannot be demanding or condescending. He is still a man and I must be aware of not treating him like a child.

That is occasionally difficult to handle. When you dress him like a child, when you brush his teeth and wash his hair like a child, when you help him at bedtime and tuck him into bed like a child, that is when maternal instincts surface and you may treat him like a child.

I am brought back to the reality of his adulthood when I shave him and remind myself that children don't grow beards. There are times that he becomes more aggressive and if I reflect on my behavior, I recognize that I have reverted to the bossy mother role and it is time to again establish within myself the respect he deserves.

I suppose each caregiver has a unique situation, but for me I have found a deeper level of understanding and patience. I draw on that to help me through the difficult times and Marshall remains non-violent.

March 12th

We returned to the dental office today. Once again we faced the problem of needing to remove all his teeth. The Xray's taken at his last visit revealed that Marshall has only stubs of teeth in his upper gums. They would have to be removed before receiving a dental plate. During our consultation with the dentist I asked if they might try to find a way to create a partial plate that would go over those upper teeth. I explained that Marshall would not be able to handle extractions. It is hard for those who don't understand the problems that arise while working with an Alzheimer's victim. They have no way of relating to his fears and limitations.

The dentist did not think my suggestion was possible, but did address a more pressing problem. Marshall's dental condition involved three upper molars that, at some time, had root canals performed on them. There were severe infections in each of those teeth. He felt that the first thing that needed to be done was to put him on an antibiotic to clear the infections, and to begin deep-scale cleaning. We would concern ourselves about what to do after that was accomplished.

We left there today with a prescription for the antibiotic, and Marshall's lower teeth had been cleaned. We will return for the upper teeth cleaning. The long period of time that visit took was enough for Marshall. He was anxious to leave.

March 14th

Linens and clothing have been disappearing. Hand towels,

washrags, underwear and handkerchiefs have been reduced to very few. Many good articles of clothing are missing, too. Marshall's "Member's Only" jackets, that were four, are now only two. It has become clear that he is throwing things away. Of course, he will deny it if questioned, but when I checked the wastebasket in his room I discovered hand towels and handkerchiefs among the tissue and waste products. I then went out to the large black trash container, that is almost as tall as I am, and looked inside to see white fabric among the waste. Because it is too high for me to reach into I opened a wire hanger and fished out an undershirt and a pair of pajama bottoms, while hoping that no neighbor could see what I was doing. It must have been a strange sight.

I'm aware that he really doesn't know how to separate clothing from trash, but the challenge remains. We need the washrags, clothing and hand towels, and I need to find a solution.

First I purchased a tall round wicker basket with a lid that would do as a hamper and lined it with a plastic kitchen bag that contains a deodorant. I placed that in his bathroom and then I asked that he put all soiled things belonging to him into that basket.

"Everything you wear and everything you use needs to go into this basket." I explained, "I don't want you to put anything in the trash because I am afraid that you might fall over the outside steps and hurt yourself."

"That's a good idea," he said, nodding his head to signal his consent.

It took some patience, but he did comply with the request. In fact, he complied too well. Today I discovered that the basket also contained his used and soiled toilet paper. It is a case of "ask not, lest you receive." Still, there is a solution for that too, and I found myself walking out of his room, swinging the dirty trash bag and humming the song from "Gigi" with my interpretation. "Thank Heaven for Rubber Gloves."

March 17th

I'm having difficulty understanding what he is trying to say. Today he wanted to have me help him find his pad. It took time for me to understand that he meant his gloves. He seems to know what he wants to say, but the words come out wrong. I must become an interpreter for his new strange language.

Most often I need to question him in order to arrive at what he is trying to express. This morning he said that someone was wandering around the house.

"Is it a man?" I asked.

"No, it's a woman."

"Someone in the family?"

"I think so."

"Does she live here?"

"I don't know, but she comes here sometimes. I think she lives far away."

That could only mean Robin, or Esther, our very dear cousin who lives in Los Angeles.

"Is it our cousin, Esther?"

"Yes." Problem solved. Of course, Esther wasn't wandering our house but she has been here often and is truly part of our intimate household.

Another time he has said, "I need my flashlight."

"What do you need it for, Dear?"

"I want to cut my hair." (He wants a scissors.)

"No, Honey, I'll take you to a barber later and we'll have your hair cut there. Okay?"

"Okay."

I know that this phase is very frustrating for both of us, but there doesn't seem to be any answer other than patient questioning. Eventually we work it out and he is relieved when I understand what he is trying to say.

Oh! My brother, would that I could move back the hands of time and have you for a little longer the way you were.

March 20th

Esther did arrive today. One of her wonderful visits. I believe this time she came to make sure that I'm all right. I know that she is concerned about what I have to face each day. She's aware of the laundry, the beds, the stress, the medication, the Ensure, the answers to questions that I don't understand, the shaving, the bathing, the late nights without time for myself, and my repeating that I can still handle it.

She makes my days easier whenever she is here by taking care of household tasks and relieving me of the chores of grocery shopping, picking up prescriptions, emptying waste baskets and loving Marshall and me very much. Marshall is always easier to be with when she spends time with us. That's normally true whenever anyone comes to visit.

Esther has been here often enough to recognize the depth of his disease and the loss we are all facing. I know that she must go home tomorrow, but I shall miss her. Marshall will not, because Marshall will not remember that she was here.

March 22nd

We had an early dental appointment this morning. That was by my request. I felt that if we had the first appointment of the day, Marshall would not have to wait as long. From now on I will try to get that first morning appointment or the first appointment after the lunch hour. Unless it is urgent, I will delay, because I feel that those appointments provide Marshall with faster attention. That may avoid the frustration he feels while waiting for long periods in a medical office. But this morning I found that getting him, Nicky and myself ready to go was really difficult.

I have never been an early morning person. It seems to take me time to generate my mind and my body. So by the time I fed our dog and let him out, prepared Marshall's morning shake and waited until he drank it, it was too late for me to have breakfast. That also meant my not taking the morning medication that has to be taken with food. Oh, well! I decided to take my meds with me and would figure something out later.

I thought it would be pleasant to take Nicky along today. The early morning suggested that it would be a cool day. There is a parking area, in front of the clinic, that is shaded so he should be comfortable if I have to leave him. Marshall really enjoys having Nicky in the car with us. While I am driving they stay close together and Marshall lovingly talks to the puppy. Nicky is definitely a calming influence.

When we got to the clinic I went inside with Marshall. He was immediately taken in for the additional cleaning. I decided then to drive through the fast-food restaurant on the corner and order my breakfast. Before leaving I stopped at the desk and explained where I was going and left my cell-phone number with the receptionist.

"Marshall is uncomfortable when I'm not with him," I explained to her. "I will only be a few minutes, but if he is asking for me, please phone and I will return at once."

The call came just as I returned to the dental parking lot. "He's getting pretty upset," the receptionist informed me.

"I'm at the parking lot," I explained. "I'll be right in."

I went at once to the room where the hygienist was working on his mouth.

"What's wrong, Buddy?" I asked.

"It's time to go home," he replied. The hygienist looked at me with concern.

"It's all right," I told her, and then focused back on Marshall.

"Just a little longer and you'll be finished," I said. "Just be patient, Dear," I urged him and wondered if I was asking for the moon.

I then explained him, "Remember that we have Nicky in the car, so I must stay with him. But I am parked right outside the door. I will be able to see you when you are finished here. Then we can go home."

"All right, Buddy?" I asked.

"All right," he replied reluctantly. I smoothed back his hair, touching him gently while letting him know that I would be near. Smiling at the hygienist as she returned to her task, I left the room wondering whether my Egg McMuffin was still warm and more important, whether Nicky had gotten a hold of it.

Nicky was fine, the coffee was lukewarm and the Egg McMuffin was edible. I also took my morning medication. After I finished eating, I put on Nicky's leash and we walked back and forth in front of the glass door of the lobby until we saw Marshall. I motioned to him to come outside and the three of us returned to the car. As I pulled out of the parking lot, Nicky lay across Marshall's lap and I heard Marshall say, "That's my little sweetheart."

Marshall won't remember what happened today, but it went well and the three of us were peaceful when we reached home.

March 26th

It suddenly has occurred to me that I often refer to Marshall as a soft, sweet man and in many ways he is just that. But he also is very human and is likely to express anger when I least expect it. Then it is either with withdrawal or sharp-tongued sarcasm. I have no defense for either. I'm very uncomfortable with his silent treatment and become tongue-tied when I'm hit with sarcasm.

Marshall's lack of patience can also be a problem, as well as his need to make all decisions. It is not that he is unkind, but he quietly needs to be in control and that includes where we eat.

When we went out for dinner has always been his decision. Where we went was also his decision, but handled more subtly. I recall many times, while he was still driving, that we would get in the car to go out for dinner.

That's when he would ask "Where do you want to eat?"

"Maybe Chinese," I might suggest.

"No," was his usual reply, "We just had Chinese the other night."

"Huh!" my mind would silently say, "That was three weeks ago."

Marshall then would continue with something like, "How does Mexican sound to you?"

"Fine," I'd reply. It really did sound fine and I never cared where we ate. I also always knew that if I had said "No" to Mexican, he would have been considerate enough to find another solution. Most important to him was that the restaurant was his idea.

So my dear sweet Brother (and that he is) is the most stubborn man I have ever known. Also the least flexible when he has formed an opinion. Add that to impatience, quiet but effective controlling and a hidden anger that is seldom revealed and you have the perfect strong silent male.

I know the games we play. I know that I have a choice in participating in those games. I also know that what I choose is exactly what I want. It is having my brother with me.

March 29th

Bruce arrived today. It seems that he and Debby have decided to give me a day of respite care as often as they can. Today was one of those days and I was looking forward to some "alone time."

It is interesting that Marshall never fails to recognize Bruce. When he walks in Marshall brightens. They play off of each other with their wittiness and their cunning remarks. They are like two boxers in a ring, and the blows are very funny. I am often astonished at how well Marshall responds with clever jibes of his own.

I wonder if all that happens because Bruce does not consider Marshall as being anything other than the uncle he has always known. It seems that all others, including myself, are aware of Marshall's deterioration. Bruce ignores it. They verbally jab at each other and often laugh together at some particular remark. It's wonderful to hear, and I love the way Bruce shows his love and affection for his Uncle Buddy.

After Marshall was in bed this evening, I asked Bruce about his approach to Marshall. "My main objective with Marshall," he said, "is to keep him alive as long as he is alive. I do that by injecting levity, lightening things up and using benign sarcasm. I poke fun and he gets that Marshall look. Then, with a twinkle in his eye, we're on our way. I'm keeping him on his toes, keeping him thinking and I'm not emotionally involved. If I don't make a joke of it, I'll get very depressed."

It made sense when I thought about it. We were watching a television movie this evening and Marshall said, "That's a stupid movie."

I would have turned to another channel. Bruce jokingly said, "Go to bed, Marshall." Marshall's response was a chuckle and he continued watching the movie.

Both he and Bruce have a dry, subtle wit. On the other hand, I am too serious. My son has occasionally reminded me that I do not have a great sense of humor. He's right, and I wish he was wrong. I would love to be able to handle Marshall as brilliantly Bruce does.

CHAPTER EIGHT

April 2001

April 2nd

Marshall is having a difficult time dressing. I never realized how many decisions had to be made while getting dressed or how many steps were needed. I'm suddenly aware of how often I look in my closet trying to decide what to wear, what to combine for the right outfit or what colors might match. It is time consuming and thought provoking. It also has become clear that putting on my undergarments, or my shoes, or my belt buckle requires some dexterity.

That explains why the steps Marshall needs to take while dressing have become physically difficult for him. His fingers don't work as they once did so buttoning his shirt or tying his shoes has become an almost impossible task. He can no longer coordinate colors, will frequently put things on backwards, and may not know that what he is looking at is a sweater. Finding things in his closets and getting dressed has become a real issue for him.

The closets in Marshall's room cover an entire wall. They are filled with items that he will no longer wear. There are beautiful dress shirts meant for occasions that he will no longer attend, handsome silk ties to complement those shirts and many pair of slacks that are too tight for him now.

It seems unreasonable that he can't wear the slacks simply because he has shrunk three inches. But body shrinkage causes the stomach to extend and the waist to enlarge, and what fit beautifully a year ago when he was taller, cannot be buttoned across the waistline now. I understand that problem. I too, have shrunk many inches and I have found things in my closet that I am unable to wear. What has been true for me is now true for my brother.

A shopping trip was in order again, but this time I took him with me. I wanted him to be involved in selecting some of his own clothes. I believe it is important that Marshall does whatever he can do. I hope that keeps him more in the present, and possibly, more aware.

We purchased three pair of slacks that have elastic waistbands. He can pull them on easily and will not have to be concerned about fastening a belt. He wanted black and beige slacks, and allowed me to buy another in soft blue. Then we went to the shoe department and purchased a pair of black and a pair of tan shoes with Velcro fasteners. He saw some shirts he wanted that pull on over the head, but I suggested that we buy only one. His closet is full of button-down shirts in a variety of colors, and I have read that it is much easier for him to wear the button type. The explanation was that a pull-over can add confusion and covering his head might become frightening. So we settled for one.

When we returned home he immediately went to the bathroom. When he came out he had taken off his slacks and was only wearing his protective underwear. He walked over to the bed where the new black pants were laying. He picked them up and I asked, "Do you want to wear those?"

"Yes," he answered.

I helped him into them, in spite of the fact that we had just put on a clean pair before we went shopping.

That brings up another condition. Marshall now changes his clothes many times a day. Occasionally, it is because he has wet them. But very often there seems to be no reason that I can understand. Apparently, he has a reason, and this most fastidious brother of mine will appear with several shirts, one atop the other, and slacks that are put on backwards. I ignore the shirts. They just don't matter. But I do suggest that he turn his slacks around because it may be more comfortable and he can get into his pockets easier. I help him make the change and hug him. Not because he needs it. I do. Sometimes hugs make the pain of who he has become a little easier to bear.

April 6th

Marshall has never been very communicative. I remember complaining to my children that we could spend all day together and not exchange ten words. Now that I look back to those days of no communication, I wonder if they could have been the early start of Alzheimer's. I didn't recognize a problem then. I just accepted that he had always been rather silent so there was little difference, but I did begin to acknowledge that there were changes emotionally.

It seemed that Marshall began to mimic my moods. If I was cranky, he became cranky: if I spoke sharply, he spoke sharply: if I was quiet, he was quiet. That hasn't changed. I have learned that making adjustments to my behavior has been necessary for living peacefully with him. My main objective is to achieve a calm environment for us both. (We're back to, if I remain calm, he remains calm.) Because I have always moved and spoken quickly, I had to force myself to slow down with my movements and my speech. I now speak more slowly and allow him time to absorb whatever I am trying to convey.

Marshall cannot be rushed, nor can he understand rapidly given information. He can also become alarmed if there is too much activity going on around him. My bustling around, as I am prone to do, can cause him alarm and I have found that preparing him for the necessary activity will ease his stress.

"Buddy," I might say, "I'm going to have to use the dishwasher. It will make some noise, but it only lasts a short time. If it bothers you, let me know. Okay?" He may not answer. But if his hands remain calm. I know it's all right for me to start the dishwasher.

There are several ways for me to judge what is going on with him. Much of it has to do with his body language. His hands often inform me when he's upset, or at peace, or facing a problem. Lying softly in his lap means at peace, tapping his fingers on the arm of his chair means that there is something he needs. That could be anything from a change of television channel to going to the bathroom. Clenching his fists is an indication that something is upsetting him and needs my attention. There are other ways of understanding through body language, too. Tugging at his slacks may mean that he is either wet or needs to use the bathroom and a clenched jaw often indicates that he is about to refuse something, like taking a shower. Our communication has become more visual than verbal. I liken it to visual listening.

April 8th

I have two friends whose husbands are afflicted with conditions much like Marshall's. My friend, Alice, has a husband who is very elderly and afflicted with dementia. My other friend, Sharon, is much younger and caring for her husband who is suffering from a brain tumor and losing his ability to comprehend and reason.

We often make comparisons and find that we face many of the same situations. We recently discussed the amount of "Thank You's" we receive for everything we do. A glass of water, an assist with shaving or dressing, turning on the television, each effort is acknowledged with a "Thank You."

I cannot believe, knowing Marshall's condition, that it is said with true appreciation. He is unable to relate to any needs that I may have. He cannot recognize when I am weary or just can't handle one more task. He penetrates my mind and my privacy with innocent disregard. How then can he understand that what I do for him requires a "Thank You?"

Of course, when he says "Thank you" I answer with a simple, "You're welcome," and we go on from there. But I do wonder.

April 11th

Today is my 82nd birthday. I have lived a very long time with many periods of independence, achievements and regrets. I sometimes think the song "I Did It My Way," was written for me. The decisions I have made were sometimes right and sometimes wrong, but they were my decisions and I lived them, taking the accolades and the blame. This all applies to what I am doing now. My choice is clear.

During all our years I have always known that I had a supportive, caring brother who would be there for me if I ever needed him. I will now be spending several years out of my very long life caring for Marshall. The amount of time is small compared to the years I have lived and he has earned my dedication many times over.

This is again my choice, and I wish that my family and friends were more aware that I would do it no differently. Their suggestion of placing him in a convalescent home is still unthinkable. I have explained to them that neither Marshall nor I are ready to consider it yet. I will know when, or if, it becomes necessary. But I do appreciate their love and concern.

April 14th

He is drifting farther and farther away. It's as though he was in a life raft drifting out to sea and one day I will not be able to see him any longer.

I wonder why I keep associating his decline with the ocean. Is it my feeling of helplessness when I stand on the shore and watch the violence of the waves? Is it their power and strength that makes me realize that I cannot fight back? Is it my soul deep communication with the lasting beauty and the calming sound when the ocean is quiet as the waves break upon the shore? Am I finding that as the wave recedes, he too recedes? Together they float, almost serenely, to another dimension far beyond the horizon and one day he and his life raft will be gone.

April 17th

There have been problems with his showering, but I have found ways to solve some of them easily and inexpensively.

Because he is very unsteady on his feet, I have been concerned that he might slip on the wet floor. I felt that it would be easier for both of us if he could sit while he showered. It might also solve the problem of getting water on his face. That seems to frighten him and though I give him a washrag to hold over his eyes, he still is uncomfortable.

The first thing I decided to do was shop for a flexible showerhead that could easily control the flow of water. They are surprisingly inexpensive. Then I went out to the patio and brought in a small white resin chair. It is really very sturdy when placed against the back wall of the shower. With the openings in the back and the seat, the water drains well and the chair dries quickly. Marshall feels secure when he sits in the chair because the arms provide him with something to hold onto. After the shower, a body towel handles most of his moisture. A large powder puff and baby powder handles the rest.

With my bad back condition, should I be doing all this? I don't know. I only know it is what I must do because it is the right thing to do. I will continue until I am unable to physically handle the situation. For now, I will add these efforts of caring for him to my mental "Must Do" list. Thinking about unpleasant tasks brings resentment, resentment brings anger, anger causes depression, and depression destroys my ability to act responsibly and lovingly. But my "Must Do" list keeps growing.

April 20th

I felt that Marshall had become unable to handle his fork or button his shirt because his muscles had weakened during his long period of inactivity. Today, while doing some research at the library, I discovered that was not only the case. Marshall is afflicted with Apraxia, a medical condition that occurs when the brain is unable to transmit to the muscles of the body. It causes loss or absence of motor or sensory skills. These are affected tasks that require patterns or sequences of movement.

According to the Merck Manual it is an uncommon disability caused by damage to the frontal lobes. The memory of sequence of movements that is needed to complete skilled or complex tasks seems to be erased. The arms or legs have no physical defect that can explain why the task cannot be performed. The muscles are still capable of functioning, but do not receive any transmission from the brain. There is another form of the ailment that causes a loss of ability to recognize objects or their uses.

Until today, I didn't know, didn't understand why Marshall could move his right leg forward but could only drag the left leg far enough to reach the right. That is what causes his very slow gate. I though I was helping him, while we walked, when I tried to improve his stride.

"Now, Honey," I would say, "move your right foot."

When he did, I would then tell him, "O.K. Now move your left foot in front of your right."

He would try and I would continue to encourage Marshall to perform a task that he was totally incapable of performing. I feel badly now when I recognize that walking correctly, buttoning his shirt, tying his shoes are remembered patterns that are no longer available to him.

April 22nd

Tonight brought about a new problem. He wanted to sleep in the other twin bed. Not the one that he has been sleeping in for sixteen years. The normally unused bed.

"This bed gets wet at night," he explained, as he pointed to his bed, "the other one doesn't."

I realized then that he does not know he is wetting the bed.

The bed just gets wet. It is true that I have really tried to avoid his using the other bed. It is because the one he sleeps in is protected with a waterproof mattress pad and a half sheet carefully tucked in. The other is not protected as well against his wetting.

The real problem is that he gets up during the night, goes into the bathroom and often returns without replacing his protective underwear, wearing only his pajama bottoms. That usually results in a very wet bed. In order to avoid his wet bed Marshall has recently decided to sleep on top the bedspread of the other twin bed, adding more laundry to an already full schedule.

I have been laundering his complete set of bed linens, as well as pajamas, undershirts, towels and clothing every morning. In spite of increasing the load, I believe that I can no longer prevent his using the second bed. I will have to make it acceptable for him. This is just another challenge, but there must be something that I can do to make it easier.

I recently was told that there were rubber underpants for adults through a Medical Supply facility. I'll check it out and if they are available, I'll purchase a pair. Maybe, and that's a big maybe, he'll replace them during the night. I can only try. But I am concerned. Marshall can't help bed-wetting, and he can't help his lack of understanding about why his bed is wet at night. But only an infant is unable to understand who wet the bed. Has Marshall declined that much?

April 25th

I have known for some time that I had to rearrange Marshall's closets. The problem that he has in selecting clothes is magnified by the amount of items he has hanging there. The shirts that he can't wear, pairs of slacks that no longer fit, pullover sweaters that are no longer needed, may make his choices overwhelming for him. If the unnecessary items are removed, it should eliminate some of his confusion. A smaller, more appropriate selection would make it easier for him.

I knew that I would need help. Standing for a long time or handling heavy items does increase my back pain. I phoned Blanca, who has been working in our home for many years and arranged for her to come and help me. She has become a part of our family and her every-other-week cleaning is invaluable. Perhaps the best thing is that Marshall likes her and she cares very much about him. Having her help me with his closets proved the perfect solution.

I think there are times that I concern myself unnecessarily. I had some trepidation about Marshall's reaction to my removing his clothes from the closet. But he was oblivious all the time we were working. After his showering, dressing and drinking his Ensure, Marshall settled into his recliner with Nicky beside him and watched the news station. Every so often I would go into the room and see if he needed anything.

"What are you doing?" he asked.

"Just straightening your closet, dear," I replied, and he seemed content.

Blanca and I worked without interruption. The closet is now organized to suit his needs. As we stood in front of the finished task, I was pleased that we had made it appear fuller while still offering him an easy selection. Shirts were narrowed down to those that he can wear every day. Dress slacks were gone, leaving only those that fit and that he can get into easily. His three robes, which he uses often, were readily available. Shoes that required tying were gone, and only those with Velcro, along with his easy to wear slippers, line the floor of the closet. I think it will work well.

Chapter Eight
April 28th

The clothes basket is no longer working. Not only is Marshall unable to recognize that putting his soiled garments in the basket is necessary, he no longer recognizes the basket. In fact, today I became aware that he may not even recognize the toilet.

I was changing Marshall's night underwear this morning when I noticed a foul smell coming from his bathroom. I went to look in the basket, thinking that he may have thrown in bowel-dirty nightwear. None appeared, yet the odor persisted and it did not occur to me to look inside his enclosed stall shower.

Bruce, who is visiting, made the discovery when he attempted to take a shower. When he opened the shower door he found feces lying on the tile floor. Marshall had apparently awakened during the night and in confusion used the shower instead of the toilet.

Bruce cleaned it up for me and both of us were saddened by the incident. It is one more decline for our wonderful immaculate Marshall.

April 30th

Today was a perfect day for an outing. The sun was shining, there was a soft breeze and Marshall seemed a little more receptive.

We would take the half-hour drive to Carlsbad. There the flower fields were in full bloom and I felt that Marshall, who had always loved the beauty of the fields, would enjoy our little trip. It was a trip that would allow us to take Nicky along and that would please him, too.

I recently had been thinking of those things that pleased Marshall in his life before Alzheimer's. He enjoyed vacationing and exploring new places, like art galleries and museums, and was deeply aware of the beauty of both. He also cared about being involved with his family; having his dog nearby; and music. Music was his passion. All and every type of music from Tchaikovsky to Rock and Roll, from Opera to Oklahoma. He understood and related to them all.

That is why I selected two tapes for our listening, the Hungarian Rhapsodies and a Glenn Miller tape. As we drove, Marshall was enjoying the Glenn Miller tape and seemed to recognize "In the Mood" and "Moonlight Serenade." Listening to the tape brought back memories of when we were very young, somewhere in the 30's, and Marshall coming home with a record in his hand asking me, "Have you heard of Glenn Miller?"

"I think so," I replied.

He grinned at me while he said, "Come on. You've got to hear this."

We went to the victrola (that's what they were called in those days) and he started to play. "Moonlight Serenade."

"It's a new band." he said, "Isn't it wonderful?"

I agreed. I also agreed with him that it was the best band I had ever heard. We loved the sound and became real fans. We both wept when Glenn Miller was lost during World War II.

Driving along listening to the familiar music was very pleasant, and we enjoyed the trip all the way to Carlsbad. Once there, I put the leash on Nicky and we got out of the car. We were facing the hillside where fields of Ranunculus spread in a blaze of color up the hill and across a wide expanse of land. They were planted in blocks of vibrant hues and the sight was breathtaking. Marshall was oblivious to it all. He sat on a bench with Nicky and me and didn't look up to see the spectacular view in front of us.

A short while later his hands started fidgeting and I knew that he had enough. "Shall we go home now?" I asked.

"Yes," he answered. I helped him rise from the bench and returned to the car. He settled in and became more relaxed. When I started the motor Glenn Miller was playing "Chatanooga Choo-Choo." Marshall looked at me and smiled in recognition. I felt that was good enough for today.

Listening to the music brought up another memory. I have played that tape before. Once when young Vailia was in the car with me. I was delighted to share the wonderful music with her.

"What do you think of this music?" I had asked my young granddaughter.

"It's nice," was her reply.

"That's my favorite band," I said, "That's Glenn Miller."

She looked at me with a questioning frown.

"Who's Glenn Miller?" she asked, and I was astonished.

I thought all the world knew Glenn Miller. I then realized that she could not have known about a musician who had performed fifty years ago. It also reminded me of how old I have grown.

CHAPTER NINE

May 2001

May 3rd

I had a talk with God many years ago. Probably when I saw Aunt Sadie reach an infantile condition. I ask God to please do anything He wanted to do with my body. That it was alright to make it old, sit it in a rocking chair on the porch, weaken it until it had little strength left. But, please, leave my mind alone.

He has done just as I asked. I have three stents in my arteries and a leaking valve. My back is a major concern with three new fractured vertebrae that can be very painful. I've shrunk three inches, which has resulted in a squashed up body that is difficult to dress well. But He has left my mind pretty well intact. Though I must confess that last week, after the fracture of another vertebrae caused intense pain, I looked up at the sky and asked, "Please, Dear God, I know that we made a pact. But could You make it just a little easier?"

There are times that I do wonder a little about myself. It is true that I may forget why I've entered a room or can't remember a word or name that I should know. But in general, this mind does just fine. I am eternally grateful for that. It allows me to work with Marshall, and to pray that I will know what to do as his illness advances.

May 7th

I believe that I finally understand that creative thinking is the key to remaining calm and compatible with my precious brother. I know that this type of thinking has frequently been called lying. But lying is a negative term and, to say the least, unpleasant. Thinking creatively often brings to the mind solutions, a new awareness and the ability to cope.

Much of Marshall's frustration and insecurity lies in his

knowing, and I stress the word "knowing," that this is not his home and that his family is far away. If I can devise where he lives in his mind, I can solve that problem by saying, "I know this house is not as comfortable, but we have to stay here until they finish repairing the old house."

We can then get into a conversation over the idea that we live in the big house in Mission Hills and all our family are still around us.

"What happened to the old house?" he might ask.

"There was a flood in the upstairs bathroom. I think one of the toilets broke so all the ceilings were damaged. But it will be alright after they finish."

We can then go on when I ask, "Do you remember when all the family came to our house for Thanksgiving dinner?" and we start to recall people who are long since gone.

He doesn't know that they are gone. He doesn't live in the world that I live in today. So we speak about Grandma making the best turkey and lemon pie, or Mother's spectacular turkey dressing. It keeps him occupied for a while and memories keep him thinking.

It often seems strange to me that he calls me by my first name, that I know all the things that he has done and all the places we have been, and I still remain someone who is not his sister.

May 9th

Gail came today. She had planned to stay with him while I spent a little time away from home. Instead I suggested that what was really needed was for Marshall to be taken out for a while. I'm not always able to provide him with outdoor activities that he might enjoy. There is often so much demand for my time that getting out of the house, even for a short drive, is difficult.

It was a great relief to have a family member offer him the outing that I was unable to give him. It worked well. They drove to the park and walked around for a while. Then he and Gail stopped for a little ice cream. Marshall was in a fine mood when they returned home. Something was said and Marshall laughed out loud. It's been a long time since I've heard the funny chuckle that is so much a part of him. It's rather amazing that with all the losses he has taken, his sense of humor remains. He comes up with some one-liners that are witty, rather than funny, and very bright.

Like the night that I took him driving through the neighborhood to look at Christmas decorations. I remarked about how beautiful one house was with blazing colored lights. Then I said something that I had thought about every Christmas, but never mentioned.

"I really don't understand this," I said. "It's like a fairyland, but what caused people to begin putting all these lights and decorations on their homes. It's supposed to be a religious holiday so it would make sense if they put up large stars to celebrate the Star of Bethlehem or beautifully decorated crosses or brightly colored nativity scenes. But these houses have all sorts of toys and many lights that have no religious significance at all. Where do you suppose that all started?"

"That's easy," he replied, and with his usual straight-faced attitude, "General Electric."

He still will occasionally say things that are bright and funny, and I often wonder how he has sustained that part of his brain. I love hearing his humorous remarks. It helps me to keep in touch with who he really is.

May 12th

I'm in a quandray. Periodically Marshall becomes upset

because he has no money.

We've been through the money problem many times, and though I have provided him with wallets and money, he hides them or throws them out, and the money is gone.

Now the problem has become more serious. He is getting increasingly restless and asks for money very often. In his mind it may be that without money he is unable to go anywhere. He speaks of wanting to go to his family or down to the market. With the lack of money he may be aware that he can't leave. He has not wandered yet. Would he? Should I?

I'll wait and try to divert his attention for as long as I can with, "I'm sorry, Buddy. I just haven't had a chance to get to the bank so I don't have any on me, but I'll get some as soon as I can."

Sometimes that works. Sometimes he forgets. There may be a time that it will not come up again. I'll just handle it as well as I can until that time happens.

May 14th

Today is the first time that I really feel like giving up. He has declined to a new stage and I am out of answers. That leaves me with a helpless feeling and some depression. The questions come more often. "When are we moving?" "Are you going out of town?" The interesting ones are "Who pays you?" "Do you have a business card?" "Are you going to the office in the morning?"

He seemed satisfied when I reminded him that I am part of the family so I don't get paid. Also, that we are both retired, that we don't have to go to any office and that I will just stay here with him.

"That's good" he answers. But is it good enough to calm his fear that I might leave him? That is the obvious reason for his concern and I must find ways of reassuring him.

May 18th

Another "Ah Hah !" day, I believe that everyone has a self-image. The kind of person we believe ourselves to be. I know that I have. I recall when my children were small and very naughty. I remember feeling stretched to the point of anger, and correcting them sharply with my voice raised above its usual level. Later, after the sweet cherubs were asleep, I would sit quietly feeling guilt at the way I had handled them.

It was then that I said out loud, "Just a minute here, you're

Vailia. Remember who Vailia is." Getting into my mind I recalled the self-image I had of Vailia. Vailia would never shout or rant at her children. Vailia always handled problems with firm but soft control. Vailia always lived with a half-full glass.

So what was I doing now? I had allowed myself to move into the half-empty glass phase. I was only seeing what was lost in Marshall. I neglect to see what remains and I must take a good look at that.

Last night he called, " Come here," as he stood at the dining room window. "You've got to see this sunset."

I joined him and together we watched a beautiful red and gold sunset until the sun went down. He often remarks about the pretty geraniums on the patio. Marshall's love of music still remains. He will become involved with television movies, but only concentrates on the background music. He especially delights in seeing the faces of babies on TV, saying how cute they are.

He still is Marshall, and what is left is all that I have, and I will continue to love and admire his sweet, sensitive self.

Chapter Nine

May 22nd

Today is Bruce's 56th birthday and I wanted to be able to spend some time with him. It is difficult to plan a visit with Marshall who wants to stay home, and Nicky who is not a welcome guest in my son's home. I know that my barking Sheltie and their Golden Retriever may not be good companions, especially if left behind while we go out for lunch. But today I was determined to do what I really wanted.

I don't think of it often, nor do I dwell on it, but the fact is that time may be short for me and I really want to share whatever I can with my loved ones. I'm a firm believer in creating memories, and I hope that I can leave behind some wonderful ones. Like those of remembering the happy celebration of a special birthday for Dad.

It was his 80th birthday and he delighted in celebrations. Marshall went with me while we searched for the right restaurant for the party. We were inviting all the family, plus many close and dear friends. There would be about a hundred people making a fuss over our father, and he would love it.

We found the perfect spot in Mission Valley here in San Diego. A garden-like restaurant that was set well off the highway, with ample parking and a beautiful large room decorated with plants and small trees. I began making the centerpieces for the tables. They were round Styrofoam circles, standing on decorated pedestals. Inside I placed the number 80 and added sparkle with blue and silver glitter.

Marshall worked on the guest list and helped select the invitations. We finally decided to use a photo of Dad that was taken when he and I went on a cruise. In the photo Dad was dressed in his black suit, wearing a formal shirt and bow tie. In his hand he held a champagne glass and on his face was an impish grin. It was perfect, and the words inside called the recipient to "Come Join Me. We'll celebrate together." It was a great day and has become a wonderful memory.

I know that I may be overly sentimental, but Bruce's birthday is just as important to me and I wanted to be with him. I made arrangements with a friend to take Nicky for the day. Then I dressed for the occasion, helped Marshall get ready and we started our drive to Arcadia where Bruce lives.

It's about an hour and a half drive if driving straight through, but I know that frequent stops are necessary for Marshall, so I planned for two hours. I also prepared a small bag with protective pads, a change of slacks should he need them, his medication and

Ensure. I have no hesitation about accompanying him into a gas stations men's restroom. Often they are limited to only one person at a time, so Marshall and I are not concerned that anyone might enter while we attend to an underwear change.

Today I included a book-on-tape and several musical tapes. He didn't understand the book, but seemed to like hearing the story. I took along the music to calm him should he become restless.

It proved to be a wonderful day. Spending time with Bruce, Debby and my granddaughter Lindsay, was a special treat. Bruce has always been my heart's delight. Debby is not only an incredible daughter-in-law, but also my best friend, and Lindsay charms my world with her loving ways and bright, expressive mind.

Today's outing gave me something to think about. I may be overprotective of Marshall. Being in the car or at home seems to be no different for him. He is no more involved at home than he was in the car. He stared straight ahead as he often does while sitting in the recliner. He went to the bathroom as frequently, asked the same questions as frequently and was no more or less agitated than he is at home. The advantage of understanding that is, we don't have to be constantly home bound. We are free to go out and we can stay as long we want.

May 25th

Marshall keeps losing his glasses. He has worn glasses most of his life, and squints in order to see when not wearing them. He does have an old pair that we use for back-up as we go on an eye glass hunt. Normally we can find the lost pair.

Today his glasses were nowhere to be found. I am concerned. I know that good vision is part of helping the mentally impaired avoid seeing things that do not exist and may also contribute to their not falling. Without proper vision the floor may look nearer than it is or the stair may appear higher. A false step could easily induce a fall.

I'm going to call his HMO to get a referral to an Ophthalmologist. However, the doctor will have to make some personal determinations. I don't believe that Marshall will be able to identify the letters on the examining chart, but I'm certain the doctor will understand.

I realize that it may appear too late for me to be concerned for Marshall about such things. I don't think so. I'm not having his hearing checked, though that too can be important. In some cases, lack of understanding may be confused with lack of hearing. But if Marshall's hearing is impaired, it could mean the purchase of a hearing aide that he would never wear. Protecting him visually is more logical. One fall that might cause a broken hip, would not only be serious, it would also be very painful. I prefer to have him pain free.

May 28th

As Marshall declines, I become more conscious of his personal hygiene. He sits most of the day now, and I need to watch for body sores or irritation. It is much the same as if he were bedridden.

Pressure points can become irritated. I often will place a small pillow behind his back or move his arms from resting on the side of the chair. Frequently they have been in the same position too long and the pressure needs to be relieved. When he is cooperative I will gently move his arms and legs. He sometimes smiles when I do that while I sing a little song, "One little, two little, three little Indians" in rhythm to the movements. We both think it's funny, but in the meantime he is getting some form of exercise.

I check for skin irritation each time he showers, or ask the temporary caregiver to let me know if there is any sign of redness or rash on his body. What is of most concern is a rash, such as a child might have with a diaper rash. Though his underwear is changed often, as are his trips to the bathroom, I can't manage to keep him free from urine irritating his skin. That is especially true through the night. The same ointment that I used on the children, Desitin, I find effective for controlling the rash, though it needs to be applied frequently.

I often will ask a respite caregiver to massage his body with moisturizing lotion. His skin is so dry. I also will have them clip his finger and toe nails. It's funny, I wasn't squeamish about changing and cleaning his catheter when he last returned from the hospital. I've never have been uncomfortable about changing his underwear or showering him. But I find clipping his nails very distasteful, almost repulsive. I haven't figured that one out yet. Guess I would do it if I had to. I'm happy that I haven't had to yet.

CHAPTER TEN

June 2001

June 1st

Marshall has entered the third and final stage of Alzheimer's disease. How do I know? I know because there are recognizable symptoms that allow me to understand how much Marshall has declined.

Lists of symptoms appear in many published documents, along with the length of time that can be expected for each stage. The first stage is generally recorded as lasting 2 to 4 years, leading up to and including diagnosis. The second stage is the longest stage of 2 to 10 years. The third, the terminal stage, is the one Marshall appears to have entered. It can last from a few months to 3 years.

Some of the symptoms that occur during the last stage and the ones that apply to him are:

He is losing weight, even with no change in diet.

His balance is poor, causing unsteadiness and stumbling. When he will use it, a walker helps.

He speaks very little and then only with a limited vocabulary.

There are long periods of sitting and he does not respond when I suggest going for a walk or into another room

He seems unable to understand much of what I say.

He is lethargic and unaware of his surroundings.

He is sleeping more and I find him lying in a fetal position at the top of his bed.

He stares into space and is unaware of any activity around him.

He needs my assistance for many things, including being able to get out of a chair or off the bed.

He requires full-time help with personal care, including using the toilet..

Marshall has all the symptoms that are described for last stage Alzheimer's patients. Now I live with the question of "How much longer?" And pray for time.

June 2nd

I've decided that I must do something about my back. The pain has become intolerable and I've discovered a lump that should be attended to. I have had breast cancer and in spite of the fact that I have done very well and am now eleven years past surgery and radiation, lumps do require attention. It is also possible that I've been abusing this back with tasks that require lifting and bending. Nonetheless, tasks must be done and I need to do them. Just wish I could find a way to make them less painful.

I will call my doctor to see if there is anything I can do to relieve the pain, other than not sitting for hours writing this book. The book is Marshall's and my legacy. It is my hope that the words written here will be beneficial to those who are facing the same conditions.

I also must find a way to live with the pain if there is no solution. I do know one thing for certain, being an Alzheimer's caregiver is not for sissies.

June 4th

Adrianne is no longer able to provide respite care for me. She is using all her free time to return to school. I respect her effort, but am concerned that the Alzheimer's Association has not yet been able to find volunteer help for me in my area. Although I realize that help may soon become available and that the association is using every means to provide it, I have an immediate need to find a temporary solution.

My cousin, Hymie and I have purchased tickets to attend the La Jolla Playhouse and I don't know what to do about caring for Marshall that evening. I spoke with my friend, Sharon, who has several people helping her. She suggested that I contact Rose, who she said is very sweet and gentle, and probably would be suitable for Marshall. She also informed me that Rose has a medical assistant background and had worked at our local hospital.

I phoned Rose. She sounded fine and said that she was available for the evening of the play. She also explained that she would work short shifts when I needed that assistance. I then suggested that she come over to spend an hour with Marshall prior to my leaving. That way he could become adjusted to her being with him. It should work out fine. More expensive than a volunteer, but a wonderful solution.

Chapter Ten

June 5th

Rose is a delight. There is an aura about her that expresses tenderness and caring. She's a little woman, with short black hair, a cherub round face and the kindest eyes. Though it's impossible to guess her age, it appears that she is somewhere between thirty and fifty. Marshall responded well to her soft voice and her gentle manner. She will work out beautifully.

June 8th

Facing the same unsolvable problem day after day often leads to frustration. Remaining kind becomes problematic. Going into his room and finding the bed had been made, though he has been asked many times not to make it, can be annoying. Today, the pad and half-sheet that I had placed there the night before were soaked with urine, as was his pillow (which I will have to replace today). Because he put the blanket, the top sheet and the bedspread across the wet area, they too became saturated with urine. All needed to be laundered.

It was while I began stripping the bed that a thought came to me, *God, grant me the serenity to accept the things I cannot change.* Of course, I thought, *The Serenity Prayer.*

Though it applies to many situations, I cannot think of an area where it is more needed than that of a being a caregiver. I recite the prayer to myself:

God, Grant me the serenity to accept the things I cannot change,

Courage to change the things I can,

And the wisdom to know the difference.

I have to realize that I must accept the things I cannot change. In doing so, I can also accept the Biblical saying, "follow after the things which make for peace." I have had enough mental and emotional upset about bed making; I'll now just add it calmly to my "Must Do" list.

June 10th

Another urine involved day. Marshall wet both twin beds. As I changed the first one the stress on my back brought about such pain that I walked into our family room with tears in my eyes and said to him, "I can't do this anymore."

Of course he didn't know what I meant, but I had to express that bending over was just too painful to bear. Then my normal reaction came to the fore. I have lived long enough, throughout my 82 years, to know that everything always works out. You just have to figure out how to make it happen. So I figured that, in order to lessen the pain, I would simply have to find help in the morning to assist me in caring for Marshall.

Phoning agencies didn't work. The cost per hour is prohibitive and they require a minimum of four hours. Even if I could afford the rates, I don't need anyone for four hours. I know I could call Rose. She is great with Marshall, but I need someone daily and her two-hour morning shift would also be costly.

It then occurred to me that it is summertime. High school and college students are on vacation. A few phone calls to school counselors brought about a fine young girl who lives in the area and is willing to help me at the same rate she charges for baby-sitting. Five dollars an hour is affordable.

Leslie, the young girl, was here this morning for two hours. She changed his linens, watered my little geranium garden, and emptied his bathroom hamper. We separated the clothing from the wet disposable undergarments and threw the disposable items into the trash. She then helped me with Marshall's laundry. My pain today is tolerable.

June 12th

I now have three identities. One as his sister (who he believes is working again in Santa Barbara), the other as Vail (who he accepts as a cousin) and the third as a new "little woman," who is concerned about her car and he wants to know how can he help her.

He heard me talking to my cousin on the phone and explaining that our car, the only one we have, really needs to have several repairs. Those repairs are expensive and I was attempting to find out if my cousin knew a reasonable and reliable mechanic.

When I asked Marshall who the "Little Woman" was, he replied, "Maybe you're a friend." My multiple personalities confuse me. I'm not really sure who he is talking to and at any moment I might be switched from one to another in his mind. I believe the time has come for me to seek more help with this new stage. I need to understand him, and it, better. Back to the Library, the support group and the Alzheimer's Association.

June 16th

Something has been bothering me as I write this journal. I wonder if I sound like a martyr. My normal feistiness prevents my behaving like one, but as I read my material I realize that what I am writing may make it appear that way.

The difference, I believe, is that I don't fit into the Webster's description of a martyr, "One who suffers great pain or misery for a long time." It doesn't mention anything about being tired or cranky, which I can be. As for great pain, I suppose my back might account for some of that. But it would be there regardless of what I am doing and I most certainly am not miserable. I'm simply doing what is right for me to do.

I have learned a lot during this phase of our lives for both of us and through a great deal of study I have developed ways to make each day and every condition more tolerable. A martyr, No! A saint, Of Course Not! A loving and dedicated sister, Oh! Yes! And like everyone who keeps a mentally afflicted loved one at home and cares for them through the longest "Good Bye," I know the difference between martyrdom and compassion.

June 20th

Leslie informed me yesterday that she would no longer be able to come. She was leaving to spend a month with her grandparents in Montana. The ten days that she had worked here was great help. I shall miss her,

Now I face a new dilemma. Leslie was exceptionally bright and very willing. Do I want to try training another schoolgirl or try to manage my budget with Rose? Rose required no training, was perfectly competent and Marshall liked her. I opted for Rose. It was the easiest solution for me, but I arranged for her to be here every-other morning. I'll just manage on the in-between days.

June 23rd

Speaking of controlling a temper, today was an example of my trying to perfect my patience level. It was not a Rose day and because she was not here to help him, Marshall flatly refused to shower. His attitude was that he didn't need it and that he would decide when he wanted to take one. With some coaxing, I finally convinced him that he had wet the bed last night and without a shower he would get a rash. I did not mention the unpleasant urine smell that permeated him and his clothing.

He seemed to understand that a rash would give him a bigger problem than a shower and went into his bathroom. I gave him a bath towel and wash rag, set the water at a comfortably warm temperature and left to clean his bedroom. I thought that I would try once more to see if he could sit in the shower chair and handle washing himself. It didn't matter how well he washed, only that he used enough water to freshen his body. I felt that however he showered, it would be good enough for today.

As I began cleaning his room, I was close by his bathroom and could hear him if he needed me. I have mentioned that, because Marshall needs seclusion, the master bedroom has always been chosen for him. There he has his desk, his television, his phone and a wonderful master bath with a large stall shower.

A few minutes after he had gone into the shower he came out with dry hair, wearing the same garments he had been wearing and stating that he had taken a shower.

"No, Dear" I said, " you haven't." I then suggested that he returned to the bathroom and get into the shower.

He had the angry look of a little boy stomping his feet and denying that he was lying, but he returned to the bathroom. When he came out again he had not used the washrag or soap. Obviously, he had just stepped under the shower. Just enough to get wet. I was really annoyed until it occurred to me that there might be a deeper reason for not wanting to shower.

I recalled that many patients with his affliction could suddenly become afraid of water, or because an area of the brain that controls the temperature may have become damaged, the water may seem too hot or cold. There might also be a fear of falling or of shampooing. The possible fears are numerous, as are the other causes including being embarrassed at being reminded to take a shower.

The solutions are numerous, too. My solution was to calm him by gently suggesting that I go into the bathroom with him and help with his shower and that we would not have to wash his hair this time. That worked and he was clean and smelling fresh when I helped him dress and get ready for the day ahead. Obviously, I was wrong. Marshall cannot handle his own shower ever again.

June 25th

Today I fought back tears. I've been fighting tears all my life. I was raised with five boys (my brother and four young uncles), who mercilessly teased the only girl. Mother said, "If you don't cry, they'll stop teasing. So stop crying" and I did. But this morning tears wanted to fall.

The alarm that I set last night didn't awaken me and I slept an extra hour. I needed that hour to get Marshall, Nicky and myself fed, medicated and ready to leave for Marshall's dental appointment. After we arrived at the dental office, I explained that we would no longer consider fitting Marshall with a denture. That was when tears began to fall.

Chapter Ten

I explained to the dentist that Marshall was fading rapidly and there was a real possibility that he would never wear a denture. That it would most likely be hidden or thrown out. I felt that keeping his mouth clean and free of infection was the best we could do. I told the dentist that Marshall could not care for his teeth himself. I would see that they were properly brushed, but I would also need to bring him in for periodic checkups.

At that moment I suddenly became acutely aware of Marshall's lost capabilities. Maybe verbalizing his condition brought it in to sharper understanding and made me focus on reality. Maybe it has happened. Maybe my heart is finally broken.

June 27th

Robin and her husband, David arrived today. David has not seen Marshall since he became severely afflicted and he is anxious to be with him now. David's mother died when he was thirteen, and since then he has been estranged from his father. That is why Marshall represents David's father-figure and why David needs to spend time with him.

Marshall really does not know them, but acts as if they are pleasant guests. It is strange that he can behave differently in social situations. He seems to grab his knowledge from somewhere in his brain and present himself as being less mentally destroyed by the disease. That seems to be true of many Alzheimer's victims, and visitors are often unaware of their deterioration.

That was especially true today for David. Robin has been here often enough to know what is happening to Marshall. David has not, so he said, "Mom, he's really not as bad as I thought he would be. He seems to be pretty good."

I didn't say, "Wait, David, you've only been here one day. Tomorrow you may become more aware of his condition."

I, too, will wait and not be as annoyed as I was in the early days when my family negated my concerns. I am now aware that by denying the condition of a loved one, it may be easier for family members to cope. Eventually they will understand.

June 29th

Ever since she was a little child, Robin's favorite thing to do was to be taken to the San Diego County Fair. Delightfully, their visit coincided with the event. Today I arranged for Rose to spend the time with Marshall while David, Robin and I went to the fair.

It was a great day. I got my hotdog on a stick and Robin

got her gingerbread loaded with whipped cream. Not having any fair traditions, David just enjoyed the exhibits and ate whatever pleased him. We left shortly after dark and wearily drove home. Marshall was waiting and as usual had refused the evening Ensure I prepared for him. He would not take it from Rose but pleasantly called out "Goodbye" as she left. Then he said, "She's a nice little lady."

Rose is wonderful with him. She massages his legs, has him do easy in-chair exercises and walks him around the back yard. He is content when she is with him and I wish that I could afford her more often.

After the rest of the family went to bed, I sat relaxing in a chair while sipping on my hot tea and watching television. I was also waiting for Marshall to come out to check on me, as he usually does, before I went to bed. I soon became aware that Diane Sawyer was interviewing Nancy Reagan. Nancy Reagan was talking about her life with the President and relating her experiences in dealing with his Alzheimer's condition.

She was asked by Diane Sawyer, "How many days do you say, I can't do it. I cannot get through another day?"

Nancy Reagan replied, "I just don't say that."

I loved her answer and said out loud, "Good for you, Nancy Reagan," and really meant it. To quote her again, "We learn," she said, "as too many other families have learned, of the terrible pain and loneliness that must be endured as each day brings another reminder of this very long goodbye." How true her statement was and how very sad.

CHAPTER ELEVEN

July 2001

July 1st

This morning Marshall informed me that he slept at a hotel last night and was glad to get back to this one. He is living with more confusion. Not really confusion, just more of receding from reality.

"Can I stay here a while?" he often asks.

I answer, "Of course, we'll stay here together."

"That suits me," he says.

Later today he was concerned, "I can't find my socks. Have you seen my socks?"

He was wearing his shoes and socks. It could only have been that he lost his gloves again. He is obsessed with the old black leather gloves that he wears constantly. He comes out of his room in the morning with them on and spends much of the day wearing the heavily lined gloves that seem to comfort him. They are so tattered with torn fingers and seams that I've tried to replace them with new leather or cotton gloves. He wears the new ones only once or twice, then hides or disposes of them. His old leather gloves remain constant although he frequently hides them so well that we both spend time searching for them.

It seems that he may be using the gloves because he is cold so much of the time. In spite of the warm robes and sweaters that he wears, he does chill even during our warm Southern California days. That, too, I have learned is normal for Alzheimer's patients. Their metabolism changes and they feel cold more intensely. When it is over 80 degrees outside and I need to open windows to let the fresh air in, I often bring out an afghan and place it over him as he rests in the recliner. It really is impossible to get him too warm.

A problem exists because our metabolisms are so different. I am always too warm and he is always too cold. To paraphrase Kipling, "Hot is hot, and cold is cold, and never the twain shall meet." In other words, we won't find harmony for this problem.

July 3rd

Marshall has become so frail. I look at this small, stooped man and I miss the brother I've always known. Physically he is my brother, mentally he is a strange child/man who could not tell his night underpants from the towel that he tried to put on his body.

Other strange behaviors have become more obvious. Sometimes he is in a basement. We did have a basement when we were very young. Sometimes he is upstairs. We also had an upstairs when we lived in Mission Hills.

He is living far in the past and it is very real for him. I am sadly touched as I watch the terrible futility of a lost soul trying to find its way back to a time long ago.

July 4th

The holiday has come and gone. Marshall knew nothing of it, but I remember the family picnics when the women all prepared wonderful food and we met in the park for a festive day and a fireworks night. Marshall loved those picnics. The men played baseball, the women sat on blankets chatting, and the children ran around and argued about who got the swing next.

Today we did not honor the holiday. Marshall does better when his routine is not changed. We spent the day with him trying to communicate his thoughts and me trying to understand what he wanted to convey.

As I was putting him to bed tonight, he waved his hand around the room and asked, "What are we going to do about all this?" I didn't understand what was worrying him.

"About what, Honey?" I asked.

"All those things that are in the room," he replied.

It was possible that he might be having hallucinations. They seem to accompany the brain damage that is part of the disease. Often he appears to see things that I can't identify, but I accept that they are there for him. It is less agitating for him if I acknowledge whatever he sees and try to distract him. Tonight was one of those times.

He couldn't explain what was disturbing him and I couldn't understand. To quiet his concern, I said, "Buddy, don't worry about it. I believe that all those things are going away now. Maybe they're already gone."

"I guess they are," he said. "I don't see them anymore."

I then helped him get into get into bed and reassured him by saying; "There's nothing to worry about. Just sleep good. I'll see you in the morning."

After kissing him goodnight and telling him that I will always be with him, I left the room concerned about the hallucinations appearing more frequently.

There are medications that may cause hallucinations. My experience with Marshall taking Aricept and having severe hallucinations made that evident, though I know of cases where that medication has been very effective. Unfortunately, Marshall was not one of those cases.

Because he has not been able to tolerate many medications, I asked his doctor to avoid putting him on the narcotic type drugs. I explained that if he believed it to be necessary, I would comply with his opinion. But I am afraid of adverse reactions that would really upset Marshall and I would prefer not to have my brother become a drug-induced zombie.

July 7th

I recently discovered that Secure Horizons, the HMO where Marshall is a member, allows 80 hours a year of competent respite care. Gerry, who came today to interview me, explained that the help would be able to bathe, shave, and take care of all his needs. I realize that 80 hours does not seem like much, but the knowledge of having additional help has arrived at such a perfect time.

My back pain has escalated so severely that at times it is almost unbearable. I have long been aware that I had three fractured vertebrae. They hurt, but not as badly as they do now that I have developed three new fractures.

It was interesting when late the other night I sat watching TV and a local doctor, from the University of California San Diego, spoke about a new method to relieve the pain of recent vertebrae compression fractures. The next day I phoned the Osteoporosis

Clinic where he is affiliated, and was fortunate to receive an appointment for today.

After the examination and new X-rays, I discovered that with the new fractures I might be eligible for the procedure. There is also a fatty tumor that may affect the nerves in that area. I made an appointment for an MRI test to be taken on July 10th. Maybe, just maybe, there is light at the end of the tunnel and the pain will be gone.

July 10th

I left Rose with Marshall this morning while I went to the hospital in La Jolla to have the MRI. I'll know in a few days about the results, and if I am a candidate for a Kyphoplasty procedure.

That procedure allows the doctor to take a small instrument with a balloon at the end and insert it into the fracture. This is only applicable to fractures that are less that six months old. My new ones fall into that category. After the insertion, the balloon is expanded and the opening is filled with what the doctor called cement. That is expected to relieve the pain associated with the fractures. I hope so.

After having the MRI, I stopped to pick up Marshall's

prescriptions and returned home to find Marshall asleep on the couch in the family room. Rose had showered and dressed him, but she said that he would not respond to a short walk outside or to the exercises. He sleeps more than he did. I know that is part of the last stage. Unhappily, that's where we are.

July 11th

While I was talking on the phone, Marshall decided to leave the house. I didn't hear him. I panicked. It was frightening to run through the house calling him and receiving no answer. I looked everywhere, including inside the closets where I thought he might not know how to open the door from the inside. I was about to call 911 when I discovered the front door was unlocked. Marshall had gone outside. I quickly got into my car and began searching for him.

One problem is that our home sets on the crest of a hill. Every direction that one could walk is either up or downhill. Marshall could possibly get down. No way could he come back up.

I drove down the four blocks to a heavily trafficked road and he was nowhere in sight. I was praying and crying as I turned right and continued to the next corner. It's one of the busiest intersections in our community. He would no longer know how to follow the street lights commands. "Dear God," I prayed, "Please let me find him. He can't handle this alone."

I turned right toward the market that I thought he might be trying to reach and saw him wandering around in the corner gas station. "Thank You," I whispered as I drove to the curb and called him. He entered the car with no emotional response and we drove home.

I didn't scold. It would accomplish nothing. I simply asked him if he was all right. He said he was, but was tired.

"It's Okay, Buddy," I said, as we entered the house. "I'll help you lay down on the couch. You rest a while."

As soon as he was settled I phoned our handyman. I informed him that every door in our house needed locks that must be opened from the inside with a key and I needed them quickly. He said he would come tomorrow afternoon and find a way to accomplish what was needed to keep Marshall safe. That means that we need protection for our front and kitchen doors, and the two sliding glass doors that lead out to our very large back yard.

I'm more aware now that he is becoming angry and belligerent, and I am very concerned. I'm afraid that I may lack the ability to understand and handle this new and awful phase. He has become verbally combative, and though I hate confrontation, I am facing more of it each day. I find myself struggling to remain calm and patient.

July 12th

We woke early. I helped him dress, gave him his orange juice and began preparing his Ensure. He opened the sliding glass door and walked out into the back yard.

I asked "Where are you going, Honey?"

He replied, "I don't have to tell you. I can do whatever I want."

Staying as calm as I could, I replied, "I'm just fixing your breakfast. That's all."

"Well," he said angrily, "I have the right to do anything I want to do," and walked into the house, opened the front door and left.

I knew better than to try to stop him physically. For the first time in my life, I was afraid of my frail and very angry brother.

I phoned 911 and explained that because of his condition this was an emergency. They replied that someone would immediately be on the way.

I followed him in my car to make sure that he was safe, all the while being terribly frightened that he might try to cross one of the busy streets ahead. It was when I saw the police car turn the corner and head his way that I breathed a sigh of relief.

The officer brought him home. Marshall didn't seem angry at my interference. He came in and sat in the recliner. I prepared his Ensure, then waited impatiently for the handyman to come and change the locks.

July 13th

Marshall is safely locked in and the house feels like a prison. I carry with me the keys to the front and kitchen door, and there are locks at the bottom of our sliding glass doors that would be too difficult for Marshall to open. If I have no pocket, I wear the keys on a chain around my neck.

He was feisty today and though I needed to water my geraniums and small flower garden, I was afraid to unlock the door while his mood was so ugly. It was then that I realized that

I was in prison, too.

I have to accept that my action to lock up the house was necessary. His getting out and roaming the streets would escalate his fears, as well as place him in danger. He could never find his way home because he doesn't know where home is. As for me, sleeping at night would be impossible if I didn't know that Marshall was safe.

Marshall tried the doors several times today, found them locked, and though he seemed to have no reaction, he continued to be feisty. To relieve some of his stress, I would like to have taken him for a drive, but I just wasn't able to trust that he might not attempt to get out of the car. Instead, we watched television together and I tried to have him talk to me.

I noticed that he was looking at a picture of our mother that I keep placed on the mantel.

"Are you thinking about Mom?" I questioned.

"Yes." He replied.

"Do you remember taking her to Mayo Brothers?" I asked.

"I took her there and a lot of other places, too. But she's doing fine in spite of her condition." That ended our conversation.

Later I gave him a hug as I helped him get ready for bed, told him that I loved him and that I was so happy that I could be with him. He sweetly said that he was happy, and he loved me, too. I hope so.

July 14th

He continues to check the doors, finds them locked and walks away. He no longer is displaying any signs of anger. I believe that the past two days were his last effort to express his independence.

It was as though he was making one more stand to protect his manhood. Trying to be who he was. Though I know he can never be again, he does not know that and it is painful and sad as I watch him fight to keep himself.

July 21st

Bruce arrived last night. He came to give me a day's respite, to let me get out of the house for a while. It's a sweet thought, and though I appreciate it, I couldn't explain to Bruce that I really didn't want to leave the house and lose spending time with him, too.

When he and Marshall came into the kitchen for breakfast, I set the French toast, eggs and butter-fried pineapple slices on the table. It had always been one of Marshall's favorite breakfasts, so I set a place for him, too. Just in case he would be tempted to eat.

He did eat and I was so pleased. After the dishes were done Bruce said, "Get out of here, Mom. Go to a movie or something. Remember, I have to leave by 5:00."

I knew he had a 7:00 o'clock meeting tonight, but then it was only midmorning and I had several hours to do with as I pleased. What I pleased was to drive out to Carlsbad, a beautiful city that touches the ocean and has an elegant outlet mall. I wandered the mall, ate lunch and tried on a few things that didn't fit. I bought some hand towels at the linen outlet store, indulged myself with a new runner for the dining room table and stopped to sit and enjoy the world and the people strolling about me. I love window-shopping and people watching, and though I accomplished little there was an inner sense of quiet and peace. I drove home refreshed.

July 22nd

I've often expressed what a sweet and gentle person Marshall is. I also explained that he probably is the most stubborn and inflexible person I've ever known. Today was a shining example of both stubbornness and inflexibility.

It's Sunday and we both slept in later than usual this morning. I woke first, let Nicky out, fed him, put on the coffee and sat quietly for a few minutes to wake up and be able to function for the day ahead.

I never know what the day will bring. It could be pleasant and peaceful, like reading the Sunday paper and leisurely scanning the ads for weekly specials. Or it could be difficult, with new challenges and attitudes. Today it would turn out to be very difficult.

Marshall seemed placid enough until after he sat down for breakfast and ate a little food. Because Marshall had eaten breakfast with Bruce yesterday, I thought that he might be ready to eat breakfast again. I obviously was wrong and know now that I will just have to keep him on the Ensure.

After breakfast he went into his room and eventually came out wearing only black shoes with no socks, a short sleeved shirt and Depends underwear. Not a pretty sight, but more importantly, not an appropriate sight.

"Please, Buddy" I asked "Go back and put on your slacks." He refused.

"I don't know what difference it makes," he said angrily, "there's nobody here but you and me."

"I know there's nobody else here, but it's not right. You don't see me running around in my underwear, do you?"

"Well, this is how I'm going to be," he stated, and sat down firmly in the recliner.

I decided that I did not have to tolerate the situation. When he asked me, "Are you going out today?" I said nothing.

"Why don't you answer me?" he asked.

I explained, "Marshall, you have a right to do as you please and I have the right not to be involved with something that I don't like. Therefore, I refused to answer a question or remain in a room with an undressed man."

"I will go into the computer room now," I said, "I have some things that need my attention. When you are ready to dress properly, I'll come back out and we can spend some time together."

I left the family room, went to the computer and waited. The time came and went for his next Ensure, but I felt he could survive without it. After three hours, Marshall walked past my door with a pair of slacks in his hand. I waited a few minutes and then joined him in our family room to find him wearing the slacks.

We spoke pleasantly to each other. He said he was sorry and I whipped the Ensure with ice cream and a banana. Then I turned on the TV and we watched our video tape of "Oklahoma."

The same situation occurred later in the afternoon. Once again I left the room and waited until he decided that my company was worth while. It wasn't as long this time until he decided to be properly dressed.

In the evening I said to him, "Buddy, I want to keep loving you and caring for you. I want to be here with you for as long as you need me. But I can't without your cooperation. Please try."

He answered, "You don't cooperate either."

Wasted effort and I wonder what new challenge tomorrow will bring.

July 25th

Watching Marshall's decline is sad beyond words. It is second only to burying a loved one. He is fighting for his life and doesn't know it. It is reflected in his fighting and defying me.

"Who told you to give me Ensure?" he'll ask. Or "How do I know you know what medication I need? Who told you what to give me?" Perhaps the worst is, "I'll not do anything until I hear from my sister and she tells me that it's Okay."

I can no longer call him on the phone pretending to be his sister. He somehow is now aware of my calling when I am away from the house and identifies my voice as the voice that is not his sister's. So I must use Dr. Joswig's name many times a day as the authority.

"Who told you to give me that drink?' I was asked again today.

My reply was, "Dr. Joswig had me speak to a Nutritionist who said it was the best thing for you. Dr. Joswig agreed. That is why I prepare it, Dear. It's to keep you healthy."

Frequently he'll say, "I'll just wait until I hear from my sister before I take that." I then explain that his sister is working and is on the road so much that we don't have a phone number for her. "But," I continue to explain, "I did talk to her the other night and she said you needed to take what the doctor ordered."

"Oh," is the answer and we've settled that problem for a while.

July 27th

It's late and I can't sleep so I'm writing this after my return from urgent care. I went there because tonight I fell and broke my nose.

Marshall, Nicky and I had just come back from a drive and a quick stop at the market. I had driven into our garage and closed the garage door. Marshall and Nicky got out of the car and were standing nearby when I tripped and slammed, face first, into the washer. I still find the fall unbelievable. I've walk over that step for almost 17 years.

Our garage, like so many others, has a raised area at the back for the washer and dryer. My opened-toed shoe became caught at the edge of the small step and I was thrown against the washer with amazing force.

Blood was everywhere. On the floor, on my dress and hands, and on the packages I was carrying that prevented me from protecting myself with my hands. It hurt and I was dazed when Marshall asked, "What can I do?"

"Call 911," I sobbed, "Hurry."

"How do I do that?" He really didn't know.

"Forget that," I said, "just go into the kitchen and get me a towel. I need to get something to hold over my nose and try to stop the bleeding."

He left and my thoughts became clearer, but still I was unable to get up. Helplessly, I waited for several minutes until Marshall returned carrying his bedspread. I realized then that whatever needed to be done I had to do myself. He just couldn't understand how to help.

So I got a towel to hold over my face, put Marshall and Nicky in the car and drove to Urgent Care. They packed my face in ice, verified that the nose was broken but that it did not affect the septum, and that I would probably have very black eyes for the next few days.

Marshall went in with me while Nicky stayed in the car. He remained detached during the long wait and was not involved at Urgent Care or when we returned home. That was such a far cry from my considerate, normally very concerned, brother. It didn't hurt that he couldn't help me, it hurt that he couldn't relate.

I have him safely tucked into bed now. My face hurts and I have discovered a lump on my forehead that is tender to the touch. It seems that I must have landed on my left knee. The whole leg hurts. If it's not better in the morning I'll have it checked.

Thank God, Buddy and Nicky are fine, so I think I'll just go to bed and take care of whatever tomorrow brings, tomorrow.

July 28th

I saw the orthopedic doctor who X-rayed my knee, assured me that it was not damaged, just a bad bone bruise, that I had no concussion, but agreed that I looked terrible. No amount of make-up could cover the incredible black eyes and cheeks.

Oh! Well, this too shall pass and I'm really all right, though I've suffered a scolding from young Vailia who demanded to know why I didn't call her immediately. I promised I would the next time something like this happens, hoping that there will never be a next time.

July 30th

Robin arrived today. What a joy! I will have her with me for the whole week and that is so special. It is rare that she can come to San Diego to be with her Uncle Buddy and me.

She lives in the White Mountains of Arizona. With the help of her husband, David and my grandson, Tavis, she is raising six children with special needs. Most of the children have been placed in her care right from birth. Leaving these precious little ones is always difficult. But she said that she wanted to be with

Marshall while he was still somewhat aware.

I'm certain it's true. By the same token, I think that she is also here to check on me. I have lost a great deal of weight and I think that the whole family is concerned. I don't know if she believes me when I tell her I'm fine as we speak on the phone. I am, in spite of the back pain and the heart condition and the amount of effort that is required for taking care of Marshall.

I have lived with back pain much of my life, also with heart problems, and I've done very well. I cannot complain about each new ache or pain, and I certainly don't want to become a complaining old lady. Most of the physical difficulties I can handle, so I place little concern upon them. The other tasks that I face in caring for Marshall, I must do and will continue to do as long as I can.

I do treasure the concern and love that I receive from Robin, David, Debby and Bruce. Those are my blood and adopted-by-marriage children, and they bring me joy beyond words. I'm lucky to be their Mom.

Marshall's Journey

CHAPTER TWELVE

August 2001

August 1st

I woke up knowing that the days seem to flow into each other. Yesterday was the same as the day before that and the day before that, and so on. I wake each morning wondering if it will again be the same, or if there may some new challenge for me to handle. There will always be slight changes, but our existence remains pretty predictable. Marshall's bed will be wet. He won't want to get up, he won't want to shower or change his underwear and he won't want to drink his Ensure. He definitely will not want to get out of bed.

There is something exhausting about predictable days. They sap your energy, both mentally and physically. The excitement of doing something new, even if only a new recipe, stimulates your interest and increases your ability to be creative and find hope. Hope that everything you do will turn out just fine, hope that tomorrow may bring a pleasant task, hope that a smile and warmth and love can be a part of that day. The repetitive day flows as slowly as the grains of sand in an hourglass.

These are the days that I sometimes wonder what I wish for Marshall. That's a hard one.

I wish him not to get any worse. I wish him to remain exactly as he is. Do I wish him not to have to live through more of this? Is my wish for him that he leave this world before he becomes an emaciated infant. Yes. No. I waver between my wishes and only know that I don't want to lose him.

August 5th

There are many times I have to make decisions for Marshall. No matter what the question, his normal answer is "I don't know," and I am aware that he really does not know. The question has not penetrated his mind. He can sense that have I asked him something, but he does not understand what it is and cannot find an appropriate answer.

This may occur when we're wandering the food court at the mall and I ask, "Buddy would you like a root beer?" I most likely will receive the "I don't know" answer. That is when I say, "Well, dear, I think you might enjoy a root beer."

Even another "I don't know" does not interfere with my getting it for him. He does like them and will probably drink it, as well as eat a few bites of the sandwich I share with him.

"I don't know," only means that he can't answer. I try to avoid questioning him as much as I can. He cannot make decisions any longer and I wonder if I always make the right decision for him. Maybe. Maybe not, but I try.

August 8th

I attended the Alzheimer's support group today. One woman informed the group that her afflicted husband had died since our last meeting. We knew that she had placed him in a nursing home several months ago and that she had been struggling with her conscience over that decision. I told her, during a pervious meeting, that we realized that placing him in the convalescent home had not made it easier for her. I explained that I had read an article saying that placing a loved one in a facility was more stressful than keeping them at home.

It really had been a necessary decision for her because he was falling. Her husband was a very heavy man and she was unable to lift or help him. Once he was in the home, she visited daily and spent many hours with him. She would put him in a wheelchair and take him outside where they could sit under a tree in the courtyard. She stayed with him while he had lunch and assisted him in his eating. She brought music and videotapes for them to share. Still, she confessed that in spite of her being with him so much of the time, she always returned home with guilt and exhaustion. As a group we really understood her pain.

After she announced her husband's death, one of the group members said, "I'm so sorry, but you must feel some relief."

"I don't know what I feel," she replied.

I understood her not knowing. I had read, in a Hospice newsletter, that grief can become more intensified a year or two after the death, but initially there usually is some numbness.

Thoughts of not having to endure the same pressures that you have known for many years might appear very welcome. The reality of being left behind without a soul mate or a dear family member has not yet emotionally occurred. The loss is too soon to feel the empty place in your heart.

During the first year after death reminders such as birthdays, anniversaries, holidays, all increase the grieving. Going through the grief period is a long hard path that will eventually come to a more comfortable end, but it takes time.

During the conversation, a woman sitting next to me said, "Vailia, won't you feel relief when Marshall dies?"

"No," I was quick to reply, "I'll keep him for as long as I can, whatever his condition. Losing him will be harder for me than what I face in caring for him."

As we left the building, one of the members of our group said, "Vailia, I want you to know how much I admire you. I think you are remarkable for all that you're doing for your brother. Not many sisters would do that."

I thanked him and wondered, "Why Not?"

I suppose that there are siblings who have separated for whatever reasons, just as there are spouses who have divorced. But the true bonding of marriage, or the true bonding of bloodline, is basic. Nothing separates you from years of devotion, shared experiences or the common bond of love. Nothing but death and that is as true for a sibling as it is for a spouse. And, in my mind, the responsibilities remain the same. I am not remarkable. I am his sister.

August 13th

An annoying day. It all began last night when Marshall once again wanted to sleep on the couch. As I explained to him many times before, I once more explained that he was not able to do that because he was incontinent and couldn't help wetting during the night. I repeated that he was just one among the thousands of older people whose bladders weren't able to hold the urine. I wanted him to understand that it was because of the wetting that it was not possible for him to sleep there.

He couldn't absorb that information. In his concept I was just being mean. I felt frustrated but I really understood. After each of his two open-heart surgeries, Marshall was able to be comfortable only when sleeping on a couch. He did that for several months before he would get back into bed. It seems to be a comfort zone for him and I hate depriving him of that.

By the same token, it is not only to protect the couch. The main reason is that the couch he wants to sleep on is in the family room off the kitchen. That is a distance from our bedrooms and his bathroom. He often needs to get to his bathroom during the night. It is there that he might replace wet underwear and can easily find his way back to bed.

My bedroom is just across the hall from his and I can often know when he is stirring at night. If he is sleeping on the couch, I'm afraid of his waking and wandering while I'm asleep and can't hear him. It really is necessary that he remains close so that I can help him if he needs me.

But he woke up today still angry, refusing to eat or take his medication. He remained grouchy most of the day, until a little tender care on my part, and a lot of affection from Nicky, softened his mood. Problem solved until the next time.

August 18th

I am not able to write as often as I did. The period that we are going through now is different. Marshall is not only needier, there is also a change in my need to be with him. Formerly, I would respond to what he asked for. He would come to me and state his concerns. Now I must watch him to know what he wants, whether it is to go to the bathroom or simply needing reassurance that I am with him.

Because it is difficult for him to verbalize, I have to depend upon hand gestures and facial expressions to understand his requirements. Often a grimace means a trip to the bathroom. His hand, touching his mouth may mean that he's thirsty. If I stand in a doorway he may give me a come-here gesture with his hand and I know that he doesn't want to be alone. Then I go and sit beside him. I talk about our past and the people who lived there. I remind him of the visits we had and all the time I know that he understands very little. But there are moments when his eyes brighten and I think may I have gotten through. Maybe just a little, but a little is better than complete oblivion..

August 26th

Our very dear friend, Ted Padzensky, died tonight. I've mentioned his wife Sharon in earlier writings. Now sadly I must mention him.

Ted was only 66 years old. His dementia matched Marshall's mental condition throughout his illness. He was not an Alzheimer's victim. It was several earlier illnesses, plus the current brain tumor, that destroyed this man during what should have been the prime of his life. Once brilliant, he had declined into a weeping child who lived in fear and distress each day of his life.

I spoke with Sharon a short time ago, and because I cannot leave Marshall, I am not free to run to her, to embrace her and to let her know how much I care. I do understand what she is feeling. I'm certain that there is some guilt because we, those of us who are caregivers of mentally afflicted loved one's, are likely to feel guilt when they die.

We have set on a fence for so long that we may not be able to know just which way to feel. In no way do we want to lose our precious partners, yet we do not want to have them become bedridden infants. Is it a blessing when they die before the reach that stage? How can we answer "Yes" without feeling guilt?

August 30th

As I reflect over my life, it seems to me that I have been exposed to Alzheimer's and dementia many times. As a seven-year-old, I witnessed my great-grandmother acting strangely when I came to visit. She had always offered me cookies and told me stories about when she was a young girl. Her stories were fascinating. She spoke about a sister who became royalty, about the Inn her family owned that stood in the middle of a forest, and how living in Poland sometimes meant facing a Progrom where bad people could come and hurt you. She told me about arriving in America and how wonderful it was to live in a country in peace and freedom and with no Progroms.

But that day she ignored me as she sat staring into space or looking at her hands and rubbing them constantly. Because her tiny hands had dark brown spots all over them, it seemed to me she was trying to make the brown spots go away.

I had been delighted when we first arrived at the big brick house where my great-grandmother Weintraub lived for so many years. I eagerly climbed the stairs to her front door, looking forward to another visit. Once inside it seemed dark and strange and quiet. Even the parrot that she loved no longer said, "Polly wants a cracker." That was the last time I saw my great-grandmother.

A few years earlier, when I was very young, I had been exposed to mental illness. My mother and I frequently walked to the bus stop. When we did, we would pass a small white cottage where I often heard a strange cry coming from inside. Mother would hurry past and I wondered if she hadn't heard the cry.

One day I needed to know what that sad sound was. "What's making that noise?" I asked my mother as she held my hand tightly and hurried me forward.

"It's the man that lives there," she replied.

"But why is he crying?" I asked

Mother slowed down as she explained. "That poor man has a sickness that makes him go back to being like a child. Its called "Second Childhood" and it sometimes happens to people when they get very old."

I recall how strange that seemed to me. "But Mommy, has that man really turned into a little boy?"

She frowned as she looked at me as though trying to find the right answer.

"Honey," she started to explain, "his body has not become like a little boy, only his mind. It makes him think like an unhappy little boy and that's why he cries."

I recall how sad I felt for the man that was crying because he had become a child. It must have left a deep impression. That was a very long time ago, yet I still recall the little white house and the sound and the sadness.

Later in my life, I experienced years of watching the deterioration of Aunt Sadie, then her son, and now these many years of Marshall's affliction.

As I became more involved with Marshall's condition I realized that my earlier experiences could not have prepared me for the day-to-day struggle and challenges that had to be met. That each experience could only have forecast the sadness that families of victims must endure. That only by living with an Alzheimer's victim can you feel the pain of a life turned inside out by the long-term memories coming to the fore, and the recent memories being lost behind them. With the realization of what is true for them, you learn know how much of your time, patience, effort and understanding will be needed.

CHAPTER THIRTEEN

September 2001

September 1st

It has been a long time since I have been able to leave the house during the day. Marshall's need to be near me has become constant. I am very much aware that his illness has also intensified. That awareness has produced an ache in my soul. It's strangely combined with a deeper level of understanding and greater realization of my love and my need for him, too.

As I look at the frail old man that he has become, I know

that life is not always fair, it is just life - giving and taking at will. What was given to Marshall was the ability to be bright, considerate, loving and kind. The strengths given to Marshall were determination, independence, appreciation and self-assurance. The pleasures given to Marshall were the respect and love of his family, his ability to enjoy, to laugh, to create laughter and smiles, to be warmly and lovingly accepted by all who knew him.

What has been taken from Marshall is his ability to think or feel or recognize any of his gifts. As I write this, lying in bed in a room across the hall is a shell of the magnificent being he once was. In that bed is a human who is no longer capable of being angry or sad or happy or content and I don't have the answer to "Why him?"

September 3rd

Now with his condition so severe, it is obvious that I need more help. The respite care that I had received was for a limited amount of days. That ran out a few months ago. The volunteers who came provided me with the ability to do my banking, grocery shopping, library visits and having work done on our car.

My needs have changed and so have my activities. My

banking will be done by direct deposit. Many major grocery markets will deliver. I have friends who will get books for me from the library. The gas station, which is only three blocks away, has offered to pick up my car for an oil change or fill-up. Marshall's needs escalate and though Rose helps me every other day, that is no longer enough.

On the day Rose is here she maintains all the early morning efforts for Marshall. The rest of the day I am kept busy caring for him, Nicky and our home. The days she is not here have become almost impossible for me to handle. There is more to do than I am able to accomplish. I need help and I'm feeling desperate as I realize that I will have to find an answer in order to continue caring for him at home.

September 4th

Today I phoned the Alzheimer's Association. They were anxious to help, but later called to inform me that they were unable to find a volunteer in our area. I then phoned Ann Sanderson of the Caregivers Association. She was concerned and kindly explained that she would try to find a way to arrange for help. I informed her that the assistance I need now is not respite care for myself. I really require assistance for Marshall's personal needs.

Ann phoned this afternoon to say that she had contacted a home-care agency and would let me know as soon as they could provide a caregiver. When Ann called back later she explained that arrangements had been made to have a caregiver sent to my home for an interview. I thanked her, blessed her and silently said, "Thank God."

September 6th

Today I interviewed Carol. She seemed very professional when she assured me that she could bathe, dress and provide whatever assistance Marshall required. Since this is the weekend, she will start on Monday.

Marshall was unaware of her visit, but then he is unaware of almost everything. He now spends his days resting on the couch or sitting in his chair with his hands lying softly in his lap. He no longer seems to be capable of expressing any emotion.

Where has he gone, this brother of mine? Deep inside has anything remained?

September 10th

Carol came to spend four hours with Marshall. She arrived at nine o'clock. I had already given Marshall his Ensure (knowing that he probably would not take it from her) and his medication. I asked her to help him shower and dress in the clothes that I had laid out on the bed, to change and launder his linens and to call me on my cell phone if she had a problem.

I didn't receive a phone call. When I returned home Marshall was still in the same pajamas that he had been wearing when I left. Carol explained that he refused to let her help him and would not cooperate with any of her suggestions. She said that he wouldn't allow her to change his underpants and kept asking if she had seen his sister.

I didn't ask why she hadn't called me, but when she left I told her there was no need to return. I know that Marshall can be difficult, but a phone call would have brought me home long enough to see that he was attended to and I could have gone back to the library to continue studying.

I'm angry. Four hours of neglect is inexcusable. If this is professional, I think I'll resort to amateurs.

September 11th

I have been letting Marshall stay in bed until 9:00 in the morning. That is where he prefers to be. I wait until I have finished some chores, prepared his Ensure for blending, and until I am mentally alive. I am the Zombie of the family when I first wake up. It has always taken me a while to become alert and ready for the day ahead. In fact, I usually set my alarm ahead of the time I need to get up to allow my sleepy mind to activate. This morning, I opened his door, said "Goodmorning, Honey, time to get up."

"Can't I stay here?" he asks, as he now does every morning.

I think to myself that the time will come when he will stay, but not yet. He still can walk, he still can see, he still can hear, and perhaps there is some thought left. Oblivion? Not yet.

"No, Darling." I said. "You need to get up so we can change your underpants. Besides, I miss you and Nicky misses you when you're not with us."

"Okay," he says, as he struggles to get up. I hurry to help him.

After setting him on the stool that had been placed in his bathroom, I unfastened his night underwear and was struck with horror. His night pad was full of blood. I didn't know how long he had been bleeding. I didn't know why he was bleeding. I only knew that something was terribly wrong and he needed help.

Marshall saw the blood but was unaffected by it. He was also unconcerned when I picked up the phone and called Dr. Joswig's office. I may have sounded hysterical when I explained the situation, but calmed down when Dr. Joswig came on the phone and said, "Take him right into Urgent Care. They'll let me know what is going on and will call me if they need me." Because Urgent Care is in the same building as our doctor's office, I felt comfortable taking him there and being close to help if it was needed.

When we arrived they immediately took Marshall into the emergency area, put him into bed and began blood tests to determine the cause. Sitting in a chair beside his bed, I waited and waited and waited. Finally, I received the information that Marshall had a urinary tract infection. After speaking with his doctor, Marshall was given an injection, an antibiotic was prescribed and I received instructions to make an appointment with Dr. Joswig for the following day.

When we returned home, I helped him with a quick body shower to remove the blood- stains, put on his protective underwear and assisted him into pajamas and a robe. After changing his bed linens, he gratefully went into bed. The Ensure could come a little later; right then we were both exhausted. Marshall, because of the constant pressure on his body and mind. Me, because of the stress and the fear.

September 12th

Our appointment with Dr. Joswig today was for late morning. Marshall's temperature was normal and after the first episode there had been no more bleeding. I will need to continue the antibiotic and make certain that he is getting enough fluids.

I also spoke with the doctor and suggested that I might need to contact the San Diego Hospice for in-home assistance. I had avoided Hospice help because I dreaded admitting that Marshall's death would most likely occur within the next six months. The stipulation set for Hospice care is the probability of death within a six-month period.

I know the San Diego Hospice to be an incredibly wonderful and caring organization. I have experienced their concern when both my uncle and aunt died there. I watched them aid their patients toward a peaceful death, and I have received their offer of support for family members. The family support extends beyond death through the mourning period. That considerate help is available for as long as it is needed.

But, like so many others, I have avoided reaching out to Hospice because I felt it was like giving Marshall a death sentence. I was not willing to admit that he had a terminal disease that would soon cause his death. That is why I was somewhat reluctant when, later this afternoon, I phoned the Hospice.

I wasn't admitting that Marshall was dying, just that I hoped they could provide me with in-home help. After acknowledging that the doctor had approved Marshall's eligibility, I was connected with a Hospice associate, Ellen Todd. She explained that she needed to come to our home to receive additional information and verify that we were eligible for the program. An appointment was set for 7:00 p.m. on September 18th.

September 18th

This is the day I will never forget. It was a day filled with despair, fear, helplessness and hopelessness.

It began with the usual routine of my waking him, helping him out of bed and placing him on to the bathroom stool. All appeared normal until I began to change his underwear. Then I discovered Marshall had not wet through the night. His underwear and pajamas were dry, and his bed was dry. As I looked at him I realized that his face was ashen, his body very bloated and he appeared almost catatonic. Something was terribly wrong.

Again I reached to Dr. Joswig for help and again I was told to take him immediately to Urgent Care. We arrived there at 9:30 and that is when the nightmare began. Doctors and hygienists attempted to insert a catheter to release the urine and were unable to do so.

For hours Marshall lay there and waited, seemingly not aware of anything that was happening to him or around him. During the long ordeal I often went over to stand beside him, telling him that it was all right, that we would go home soon. I told him that he would feel better, that Nicky was waiting for him and all the time my heart was heavy with fear.

Time after time an unsuccessful attempt to insert the catheter was tried, and time after time I phoned Dr. Joswig's office for help in finding an Urologist for Marshall. I explained that perhaps the stent that had been inserted into the urethra so many years ago might now have become a blockage. I asked why it was taking so long to find an Urologist who could help him. I was assured that every effort was being made.

It was almost 5:00 o'clock this evening before a doctor was found to take care of him. I don't understand why it took so long. Why didn't I fight harder? As I write this I continue to question, "Why in a world full of doctors, did Marshall have to wait eight hours before receiving help?" It just doesn't make sense, and because I was so frightened and stressed I realize that my waiting and accepting the answers I received may not make sense either. It just did not occur to me to call Marshall's HMO to find out if they had been contacted and if they were doing anything to take care of the problem.

When the doctor at Urgent Care finally gave me the address to an Urologist's office he told me to hurry, that I had to get Marshall to the doctor before he closed his office. With the help of a medical assistant I got Marshall into our car and drove away. Ten minutes later, I parked the car and helped Marshall enter the doctor's office.

I had never met this doctor before, yet I could sense that he felt burdened by our problem.

Marshall was rushed into an examining room and told to get

up on the table. For him that was impossible. It appeared that he didn't understand. He just stood at the foot of the table and could not relate to placing his foot on the small step that would assist him in getting up. I stood in back of him, put my arms around him and tried to move him toward the step. The nurse lifted his foot, but he didn't move upward.

There was no use trying to have Marshall help himself. The three of us, doctor, nurse and I, lifted him up and gently placed him on his back.

I tried to tell the doctor that Marshall was afflicted with Alzheimer's but he stopped me saying, "I can see that," and then he began the lengthy procedure of trying to release the urine. He first used a child-size catheter, inserting it slowly. He withdrew that one and inserted one slightly larger. This application continued until a normal-size catheter was inserted and some urine was released.

It was then that I realized Marshall was incapable of feeling pain. He did not flinch, frown or change his countenance during the long hour that the doctor worked on him. He just lay there as though nothing was happening, and what was happening had to be painful. My heart ached for him, for his loss of dignity, for his helplessness, for his inability to feel the love and the tenderness that I felt watching him go through the terrible ordeal. Only that I satisfied his need for me to be near him made the situation tolerable.

The Urologist released Marshall with a catheter still in place. I carefully helped him into the car and drove home. We arrived about 6:30 and I placed Marshall on the couch in the family room. He seemed peaceful and I needed a few minutes to let Nicky out and feed him.

Just as I was about to take Marshall to his bedroom the doorbell rang. When I opened the door a lovely tall woman with a notebook under her arm said, "Hello. I'm Ellen Todd."

I had completely forgotten our 7:00 o'clock appointment. "I'm so sorry," I said. "It's been a rough day and I forgot about our appointment. Please come in."

She entered and I introduced Marshall. Then Ellen and I sat at the table in the family room and I began answering her questions. While she was filling out papers I glanced at Marshall and was appalled. Everything about and near him was wet with urine. Apparently his bladder had released all the urine that had remained and his pants, his shoes, even the couch and rug, were soaked.

I started to jump up to help him when Ellen stopped me. "Vailia," she said, "You can't handle this anymore. I'm going to call for our ambulance and take him where he can get the help he needs now."

It's strange, he has only been gone from the house a short time as I write this, but I cannot remember what happened from the time Ellen stopped me until I heard the doorbell ring and two attendants from the Hospice were placing my brother on a gurney. I must have been in a state of shock. All that period of time waiting for the ambulance to arrive is a total blank. This much I understood as they began to wheel him away, I had no choice! No Choice!

But I held to the thought that kept me going, that gave me the strength to continue as his caregiver. It was that he was not dying. He was just going to have them help him and then I could bring him home again. I ran over to the gurney and saw that his eyes were open, but they held no light. I stoked back his hair as I so often did, and kissed his pale, drawn cheek before they put him in the ambulance.

Chapter Thirteen

"I must go with him," I said to Ellen.

"No," she replied. "You've had a hard day and it's a long ride to the Hospice. Why don't you wait until morning when you are fresher. I promise you that he will be all right."

"But he'll miss me," I replied, "and he may be frightened if I'm not there."

"Vailia," Ellen said, "Marshall is not aware of being taken away or your not being with him. You both must rest. It is possible that he may be more alert tomorrow, but after the difficult day he's had today, he's at peace and resting mentally."

I helped her finish the forms she had brought with her. Blessed her for the hug she gave me as she left and closed the door on the first night that I will be in our home without my brother, and I'm the one who is frightened. Afraid that I may be losing him, afraid that he will want me and I won't be there, afraid that he might die without my telling him the truth about the last few years of our lives.

September 19th

After a restless night, I woke early to shower, dress, feed

Nicky and go to the San Diego Hospice. It's about a twenty-five mile drive from our home and as often as I have been there, I never stop being awed by its beauty.

A freeway off-ramp leads you to Washington Boulevard in the heart of the Hillcrest district. Driving through a bustling neighborhood of business, restaurants, medical facilities and narrow two-lane side streets, you arrive at a wrought-iron gate that opens onto a setting of incredible beauty. Flowers, arbors, trees and crafted wooden benches line both sides of the entrance to the Hospice that sets on an isolated point of a hill over-looking the valley below.

Where Marshall is now is in the Inpatient Care Center. The Impatient Center is a state-of-the-art facility. Unlike any other in the region, the Center offers quality professional, physical, emotional and spiritual care for the terminally ill and their family. As I entered his room today, I was once more aware of the compassion that is evident there. His room is light and airy with comfortable chairs and a couch that can be opened into a bed should a family member want to remain through the night. Every consideration is offered to the patient and their loved ones. I view the Hospice with almost the same sense of peace and awe that I feel when I enter a house of worship.

Chapter Thirteen

I spent most of the day at the Hospice. I brought with me some of the musical video-tapes that Marshall had enjoyed, but he didn't respond. I talked to him, stroked his hair, kissed his head, and occasionally he would look my way with a moment of recognition and a soft smile. That is when hope in my heart surfaced a little.

Late in the afternoon, when he appeared to be quietly sleeping, I returned home to feed and care for Nicky. Then I checked my phone for messages.

"Hello, Aunt Vailia," came the voice on the message machine. It was a voice that I had not heard for a long time. "It's David Schwartz. I'm sorry to have to tell you, but Mother passed away today."

I picked up the phone and returned his call. "Oh! David," I said sadly, "I'm so sorry. What a terrible loss." Not my Marie, I thought. Not the most genuine, loving, forgiving friend one could have. David lost his mother and I lost my dear friend of more than forty years.

As we spoke the memories rose in my mind. Marie and I had raised our children together. I became "Aunt Vailia" and she

221

became "Aunt Marie", not only to my children, but also to my grandchildren. We shared our religious beliefs and because our bond was so close, we became involved in each other's lifestyles.

We also looked very much alike. Marie's Italian background bestowed upon her the most beautiful blue eyes, very dark brown hair and almost Grecian features. I looked much the same, except that my eyes are brown. We wore the same size, had the same interests and thoroughly enjoyed the experiences when we were accepted by each other's religious organizations. We laughed when Marie's Catholic Guild asked me to join, and thought it was great fun when my Hadassah group invited Marie to become a member. Our children also shared our non-denominational attitudes. At Christmas, mine would go to the Women's Guilds along with her sons to sing Christmas Carols. Her boys joined my children at the Jewish Home for the Aged to entertain with Chanukah songs. Had I been able to request a sister, it would have been Marie.

David continued, "Mother insisted upon being cremated and she wanted the mass to be held here in Palm Desert. We believe that she would have wanted her ashes at Dad's grave in San Diego. So we've made arrangement for the service to be held at 10:00 o'clock on the 27th. We'd love you to be there. Can you make it?"

"Of course, Darling," I answered. "I must be there."

It will be all right for me to go to the cemetery Thursday morning. From there I will go directly to the Hospice. Marshall doesn't know when I arrive, or if I am there at all. I desperately want to be with him because it is my need. His conscious needs have disappeared.

September 20th

My back pain was so severe today that I was unable to drive to and from the Hospice. The long round trip, plus another long walk to the Impatient Care Unit, seemed impossible. I stressed over trying to get dressed and going to see him, but finally gave up when I accepted that I was having an "Oh, Dear God," day.

I've named my days so family and friends can have an answer to, "How do you feel?" They are titled "Fine" which is tolerable, "Good" which means I'm hurting some and an "Oh, Dear God" day. That day is when they know that I am leaning over a table and stretching my back while trying to make the intense pain go away. Today was definitely an "Oh, Dear God" day, so I stayed home with Nicky.

Poor little Nicky. He is aware that Marshall is gone. At night he goes into Marshall's room and waits for me to come in with Marshall and help him get ready for bed. That has been Nicky's nightly routine and he can't understand why his friend isn't here with us. Though Nicky is really my dog, we have shared our love and attachment with Marshall, and we both miss him terribly.

Nicky really has been neglected. I haven't taken him for walks or played with him for a long time, and I feel guilty about his neglect. I'm suddenly aware that I am having a lot of feelings these days. There were many times that I could analyze my feelings and solve whatever problem appeared. Now I'm just too busy and my mind is too pre-occupied. I haven't the ability to try to find solutions. I just feel.

September 21st

Marshall will not take the Ensure that has been prepared for him. The nurses and I have talked about the way I prepared it, with large scoops of ice cream in a blender. They've tried to prepare it the same way, but he will not drink. I wondered if it might be too hard for him to suck through their small straws.

On my way home I drove through a Jack-in-the-Box and ordered a sandwich and a small drink. I noticed that the straw they gave me had much larger holes than the ones provided by the hospice.

"Would you allow me to buy some of your straws?" I asked the young man at the drive through window. "My brother is very ill. These larger hole straws make it easier for him to suck through."

"Just a minute," he replied and left the window.

When he returned he had a large bundle of straws in his hand.

"What do I owe you for them?" I asked.

"Nothing," he replied. "We're happy to help." Once again, as I thanked him, I became aware of the wonder of kindness.

Tomorrow I'll take the straws with me when I go to visit. I'm going to try preparing Ensure for him at home, too. I've hesitated doing that because of the long drive, but I think it will work if I put it in a thermos. (Mother Hen! Is it because this is the only thing you can think of doing for your chick?)

I miss him so much. I miss him even as I sit beside his bed and hold his hand and tell him how much I love him. I miss him as I drive home and know that the house will be empty without him. I especially miss him at bedtime when I can no longer close the door and say "Goodnight, Buddy. I love you." And hear him answer, "I love you, too."

September 22nd

The Ensure and the straw didn't work. I tried giving it to him and there was no response.

He didn't refuse to drink. It just seemed that he was too far away to relate to the concept of drinking. I will leave the bundle of straws at the desk. It may help with others who are still able take fluids.

He is actually too far away for anything but waiting. Am I admitting to myself that the waiting is for death? Not Yet, I tell myself. He is resting here, they're taking good care of him, he will come out of this and I can take him home.

Somewhere, deep inside, I know better but I'm not ready to let it appear.

Chapter Thirteen

September 24th

Marshall is gone. I know I have said that before, but I didn't know how far "gone" was. I visit him and he does not know I am there. He no longer asks for his sister, not even to talk to her. I had said that when he no longer knew where he lived or who I was, I would consider placing him in a facility. I later added that I would consider that placement when he no longer needed me constantly and I could go to sleep without imagining him trying to find me at night. Now that he is in a facility, how do I feel?

Mixed feelings. Some despair that he is not here and a great sadness that he no longer needs me. Some relief that he is being cared for in a manner and a place that I cannot provide at home. A tiny feeling of hope and a large feeling of loss. Loss of his presence, loss of his need for me, loss of my being responsible for his care. The losses add up and, in those few moments when he was taken away, our lives were lost as they had been and will never be again.

I am on an emotional seesaw. One side of me says, "Be brave." Another side says, "It's Okay to cry."

"You never cry," I'm reminded. "You need to be strong."

I reply to myself, "I'm tired of being strong. I've used up all my strong energy. I'm going to cry."

And I do.

September 25th

My days are so full of running and driving. Of needing to do things at home, like caring for Nicky or checking the mail or writing checks. It's almost the end of the month and bills must be paid, and I don't want to think about it.

I go to the Hospice early in the day, come home to feed and care for Nicky, then go back to be with Marshall for a while. It is really that I need to be there for myself. There's nothing left that I can do for him. After all these years, that is strange.

September 26th

Bruce, Debby and Robin arrived today. I knew when they entered my home that they were here because they believed Marshall was dying. I didn't ask what their reasons were. Possibly they were here because they wanted to see their uncle for the last time. Possibly because they felt that I needed their support. Whatever the reason I was happy and grateful to have my children with me.

Chapter Thirteen

Soon after their arrival, the subject they were concerned about was brought up. It was asking what plans I had for Marshall's funeral. It was important because, by Jewish law, burial must take place the day after death, the exception being the Sabbath or a religious holiday. That requirement is what has always created early planning.

What my children didn't know is that I have been troubled about that subject for some time. I have stressed, prayed, sought direction from Rabbis and finally had reached a conclusion that I could live with. That was to have a religiously correct funeral for my brother, in spite of the fact that he had definitely stated that he wished to be cremated. In fact, he had already paid for his cremation to the Neptune Society.

As in other religions, our religious laws do not permit cremation. I had discussed the subject with my cousin, Esther, and with Robin as well as with the Rabbi's. They all agreed that since I was the one left behind, I had the right to make a decision that would be most comfortable for myself and my family. I decided to follow our religious dictates. I clearly stated to the children that what I considered a proper religious burial was my firm decision.

I explained how horrifying it was for me to think of Marshall's ashes being thrown into the sea and his being completely gone. No way to visit his grave, no stone to remind the world that this dear soul once lived here. Nothing at all left to cling to and, I explained, I need something to cling to. Robin understood. Bruce did not. I had forgotten that Bruce and Debby are members of the Neptune Society and do believe in cremation.

After the discussion, I rose from my chair, picked up some papers that had fallen on the floor and went into the kitchen to throw them away. Suddenly Bruce appeared in the doorway.

"That is the most unforgivable thing I have ever heard." He was angry. His stance and face reflected how deeply he felt. Tight jaws, hand stuffed into his pockets and glaring eyes that met my gaze.

"How can you possibly ignore Marshall's decision?" he went on. "He made what he wanted very clear. I can't believe that you would ignore that. Mom, you have to think it over. You have to decide what is really right for Marshall. What you are thinking of doing is not honoring him. If you have a funeral, I won't be there."

He turned and stomped back into the living room. I dropped into a chair feeling defeated and alone. I put my head in my hands and covered my eyes. I sat quietly praying for an answer. My son's opinion and desires are important to me. My own needs and those of my family, who more closely follow our religious concepts, are important to me. I'm lost again and I don't know what to do.

September 27th

The longer I live the more I am convinced that life if full of miracles. This morning I went to Marie's funeral and found a miracle waiting for me there. David and his brother, Richard, greeted me warmly with hugs and kisses. Then David escorted me to the mourner's tent near the grave of their father, Frederick Schwartz. I was placed in a chair in the front row close to the grave.

Then came my miracle. As I looked at Frederick's grave, I noticed a small hole had been dug there. The reason it was there did not occur to me. I thought perhaps for planting plants or flowers. My thoughts returned to the ceremony.

The priest who had accompanied them from Palm Desert beautifully conducted the service. Then he brought up a small wooden box with a lovely golden cross on top. It held Marie's ashes. After another prayer was said, the box was placed into the little hole on Frederick's grave. Mourners rose and each scattered dirt on top of the box. I sat for a moment and said to myself, "I could do that. I really could live with that."

I mourned the loss of my friend and thanked her once again, for giving me a gift that I hadn't expected. By burying the ashes, we could solve the problem of Marshall's funeral arrangements.

When I returned home, I explained to the children that there was a solution for Marshall's funeral. He could be cremated and we could have a religious funeral and burial as well. I explained what I had seen and they agreed that would be perfect. Then the questions arose.

"Mom, do you know a Rabbi who would perform the service?" Robin asked

I did not and knew that very few Rabbis will perform a cremation service. The Rabbi at the synagogue I attend certainly would not participate. Most consider cremation the desecration of a body and against Jewish law.

Again, a question, "Will we be allowed to bury him on sacred ground in the Jewish Cemetery?" I don't know, I thought. Will we?

Robin got up, "I'll make some phone calls, Mom. We'll just find out what we can do. Okay?"

"Of course," I said to my capable, competent daughter.

Two hours later Robin came into the room to tell us that all had been solved.

"The Chaplain at Camp Pendleton is Jewish and will perform the ceremony." she said.

"That's a relief," I replied. "What about the cemetery?"

"Mom," she explained, "that's really interesting. I phoned and asked if they would accept a cremation burial. The man I spoke with replied that they now have a small corner where such burials are being permitted. We could come and pick out the plot.

When he offered directions, I explained that they weren't necessary. I told him we knew where to go because most of our family are buried there.

"You won't believe what happened next," Robin continued. "That man said, you didn't tell me you had family buried here. You have the right of Second Internment. He then explained that it is permitted to have another burial in an existing grave."

I would not have believed it had I not witnessed it at Marie's funeral. I just didn't know that it was available in our religion. I do know that it is an especially appropriate solution for Marshall's funeral. Marshall will be buried with his mother. That is the perfect ending for the perfect love they shared.

CHAPTER FOURTEEN

The Journey's End

September 28th

I have been waking every morning to the awareness that Marshall is not here. I hurry to feed Nicky, let him outside and dress quickly so I can leave to go to the Hospice. I don't think Marshall knows when I am with him. There is no communication. He quietly lies there and may softly smile at the nurses who come in to care for him. They all tell me how sweet is, and I answer, "I know."

Yesterday I had phoned to ask Roger, the nurse practitioner, if they could try to get Marshall on his feet. I felt that if he was mobile, I might be able to take him home and care for him. After I arrived today Roger came into Marshall's room and we talked for a while.

His tone expressed sympathy as he explained, "We did try to get Marshall on his feet but he hasn't the strength to stand. I'm sorry."

As we talked he looked toward my brother then turned back to me and said, "You know, I've seen hundreds of patients in your brother's condition. I have never seen any whose face was so peaceful. Someone had to have taken very good care of him."

At least, Thank God, I had accomplished that much. So why do I feel that there were times I failed him? Why do I remember what I had not done, rather what I had done? Why do I recall the times that I lost patience, rather than remembering the nights that I put him into bed with a hug and a kiss? Or when I softly stroked his hair as I explained that I would never leave him alone at night, that I would always be with him. What makes me ignore the smile on his face as I reassured him that he would be safe, or his answer of, "That's good."

How deeply I wish that I could once more close his bedroom door as I say, "Goodnight, Buddy. Sleep good. I'll see you in the morning." Often I would add, "I love you." And he would answer, "I love you, too."

Tonight I could stay with him all night because my children were at my home and would care for my problems there. The Hospice offered me the comforts of a blanket and a couch to rest on. As I lay there, I closed my eyes while I listened to Marshall's breathing. I drifted in and out of sleep until, at two in the morning, his breathing changed. I heard it become raspy and strained.

I jumped up as his nurse entered the room. "Is my brother dying?" I asked.

"Yes," she replied as she touched his body. "His feet and legs are already cold. But be careful of what you say. The hearing is the last thing to go, so he can probably still hear you."

I moved quickly to his bed and leaned close to he ear.

"Buddy," I said, "I have lied to you for a long time. I had to because you could not accept the truth, but now I want you to know that your sister never abandoned you. She has been with you every day and every night. She never left your side."

His mouth, that had been hanging open, closed slightly and there was the tiniest hint of a smile in the corner. I know he heard me. I stood beside him, stroking his hair and holding his hand. Fifteen minutes later my brother died.

September 29, 2001

On this day the world may cry for his loss,

but in heaven the angels will sing for the return

of one of their own.

www.ingramcontent.com/pod-product-compliance
Lightning Source LLC
Chambersburg PA
CBHW030304290526
45785CB00001B/214